SACRAMENTO PUBLIC LIBRARY

3 3029 05327 9006

CENTRAL LIBRARY
828 "I" STREET
SACRAMENTO, CA 95814
DEC - - 2003

"Beth Ann Hill's book for MS pa[...] and practical advice. It factually and optimistically answers the most common questions asked by MS patients and steers them in the right direction when they want to learn more. It is an ideal first book to read for new MS patients."

—JAMES L. BERNAT, M.D., PROFESSOR OF NEUROLOGY
AT DARTMOUTH MEDICAL SCHOOL

"This book is well written, by and for persons with multiple sclerosis (MS), and deals clearly and concisely with many of the issues that are important at all stages of the disease."

—DR. H. MATTSON, M.D., PH.D., PROFESSOR
OF NEUROLOGY, DIRECTOR OF THE
INDIANA UNIVERSITY MS CENTER

D1021226

document is full of useful information.

MULTIPLE
SCLEROSIS Q&A

. . . .

Reassuring Answers to
Frequently Asked Questions

. . . .

Beth Ann Hill

AVERY
a member of
Penguin Group (USA) Inc.
New York

Neither the publisher nor the author is engaged in rendering professional advice or services to the individual reader. The ideas, procedures, and suggestions contained in this book are not intended as a substitute for consulting with your physician. All matters regarding health require medical supervision. Neither the author nor the publisher shall be liable or responsible for any loss, injury, or damage allegedly arising from any information or suggestion in this book. The opinions expressed in this book represent the personal views of the author and not of the publisher.

While the author has made every effort to provide accurate telephone numbers and Internet addresses at the time of publication, neither the publisher nor the author assumes any responsibility for errors or for changes that occur after publication.

Most Avery books are available at special quantity discounts for bulk purchase for sales promotions, premiums, fund-raising, and educational needs. Special books or book excerpts also can be created to fit specific needs. For details, write Penguin Group (USA) Inc. Special Markets, 375 Hudson Street, New York, NY 10014.

AVERY

a member of
Penguin Group (USA) Inc.
375 Hudson Street
New York, NY 10014
www.penguin.com

Copyright © 2003 by Beth Ann Hill

All rights reserved. This book, or parts thereof, may not
be reproduced in any form without permission.
Published simultaneously in Canada

Library of Congress Cataloging-in-Publication Data

Hill, Beth Ann.
Multiple sclerosis Q & A : reassuring answers to frequently asked questions / Beth Ann Hill.
        p.   cm.
Includes bibliographical references and index.
ISBN 1-58333-174-3
1. Multiple sclerosis—Popular works.   I. Title: Multiple sclerosis Q and A.   II. Title.
RC377.H55   2003   2003044380
                616.8'34—dc21

Printed in the United States of America
1   3   5   7   9   10   8   6   4   2

Book design by Amanda Dewey

To my sweet Savior,
who provided the contents
of this book in a dream

Acknowledgments

I would like to thank the following individuals and organizations for their help with both the writing of the book and with my day-to-day battle with MS: Sheila Curry Oakes and my editors, Kristen Jennings and Amy Brosey, for their tremendous help getting this book published; Dr. Joanne Wojcieszek, for spending so much of her time helping to edit the book and for the wonderful foreword; Dr. James Bernat, for his insightful suggestions and for being the first to endorse my book; the National Multiple Sclerosis Society for its assistance in so many ways, and particularly Arney-Ellen Rosenblat, for her guidance and help with so many issues; David Lander, for his kindness and for making me smile; Neil Cavuto, for taking time out of his incredibly busy schedule to read my book; my neurologist, Dr. Thomas Schrieffer, and family physician, Dr. Craig Bethune, for helping me with my own personal struggles with multiple sclerosis; my mother-in-law, Monna Lee Hill, for all the times she came and took care of the children so I could write, for the times she helped manage the household when I was ill, and for her many prayers; my mother, Shirley Praed, for listening to me when I am discouraged; my dad, Jack "Pops" Praed, for his creativity; my brother Jon Praed, for our special trip to swim with the dolphins; my brother Scott Praed, for showing me how to live hopefully ever after with adversity; my friends Shawn Hanson and Katie Reitemeier, for cleaning my house when I couldn't, for listening when I needed to talk, and for making me laugh; my brother-in-law, Brian Hill, for helping with the children so I could write; my long-distance friend Dona Faircloth, who always understands; my oldest and one of my dearest friends, Becky Fletcher, who always makes me feel special; my wonderful friend Jeanne Kost, who has gone through so much with me; my dear friend Stacy Parsons, for making me laugh; my principal, Maggie Antcliff, and the entire staff at Ken-O-Sha Elementary School, for their support and encouragement; my friends Noel and Kathie Griese, for believing in me; my former professor, Dr. Leonard Teel, for challenging me; and finally, my husband, Danny, the love of my life.

Contents

What is multiple sclerosis? • What causes MS? • But can't some diseases have more than one cause? • Why does MS occur? • Is MS similar to AIDS? • Can I get MS from my spouse? • What are the different categories of multiple sclerosis? • What is "silent" MS? • What is an attack? • What causes an attack? • Why do some attacks produce permanent damage but others don't? • Can stress cause an attack? • Can illness cause an attack? • What is a "pseudo-exacerbation"? • Can exercise cause an attack? • Can the nervous system repair itself after an attack? • When I tell people that I have relapsing-remitting multiple sclerosis, they ask if I am in remission. I don't know how to answer. I'm not having an attack, but I sure don't feel like I'm in remission.

History and Statistics

How long has MS been around? • Who discovered MS? • Who gets MS? • How many people have multiple sclerosis? • At what age does someone usually develop symptoms of MS? • Is MS more common in certain parts of the world? • Does where you grew up make a difference in your susceptibility to MS? • Is MS an inherited disease? • Is there an MS gene?

Symptoms

What are the symptoms of MS? • What kind of vision problems could I possibly develop with MS? • I was recently diagnosed as having optic neuritis by my ophthalmologist. Does this mean that I will develop MS? • You mentioned altered sensations in the list of possible symptoms. What kind of altered sensations are you talking about? • Do people with MS experience pain? • What is spasticity? • What is tremor? • What is vertigo? • What about fatigue? Is fatigue a common symptom of MS? • What kind of cognitive impairment problems can MS produce? • Can MS cause depression? • What kind of bladder dysfunction can MS cause? • What kind of bowel problems can MS cause? • What kind of sexual problems can MS cause? • Can an MS symptom last for just a short period of time? • What course will my disease take? • Can MS "burn out"? • Will I end up in a wheelchair? • Can MS be cured? • When do experts believe a cure will be found?

Diagnosis and Medical Tests

How is a person diagnosed with MS? • Can MS be mistaken for other illnesses or vice versa? • My doctor just told me that I have MS. I think I've had MS for years! How did he arrive at this decision now? • What are the medical tests that are used to pinpoint MS? • What can I expect during an MRI? • I've had an MRI, but nothing showed up that was abnormal. Does this mean I don't have MS? • What can I expect during a spinal tap? • What can I expect during an evoked response test? • Are there any new tests being developed to help diagnose MS?

Treatment

How can I find a good neurologist? • Which drugs are used to fight MS? • Can someone take one of these medications if they have "probable" MS? • Which of the disease-modifying medications should I choose? • My insurance doesn't cover any of the disease-modifying medications! What should I do? • Are oral versions of these drugs available? • What about combining medications? • What about Novantrone? • Can someone with progressive MS take Avonex, Betaseron, Copaxone, or Rebif? • Is there anything else that is being done for people with secondary-progressive MS? • Are there any new medications on the horizon? • Which medications are used for major attacks? • Are there any side effects from being treated with corticosteroids? • What other medications are used to treat the symptoms of MS? • What kinds of therapies are available to MS patients? • There are so many illegitimate claims of curing MS. What about alternative practices? • What are some alternative therapies for MS? • Will a special diet help my MS? • Will vitamins and minerals help my MS? • What are megavitamins? Will they help my MS? • Will medicinal herbs help my MS? • Do amalgam dental fillings cause MS? Will having the fillings removed make my MS go away?

PART III: SUGGESTIONS 87

· ·

Foreword

Multiple sclerosis is always unexpected. This neurological disorder intrudes on people in the prime of their lives. Just as one begins to launch a career and start raising children, MS interrupts plans and time lines. Patients must stop and reassess their priorities, values, and aspirations. Probably the most frustrating aspect of MS is its unpredictable course and prognosis. Every patient has his or her individual constellation of symptoms. Despite these intrinsic differences, there are some clear unifying aspects of MS that all patients share. Many patients struggle with unusual, vague symptoms for many years before a definitive diagnosis is made. The actual moment of truth, when the neurologist tells someone that they have MS, is a powerful and shocking experience. The emotional response to receiving such news can be one of disbelief and denial for some, while for others it may be relief following a long journey searching for answers.

Routine visits with the neurologist rarely include ample time for patients to have all of their questions answered, especially immediately following their diagnosis, when they may feel overwhelmed by the complexity of MS. How nice it would be to have a concise and accurate book that could answer the important questions about the disease. That is precisely what Beth Hill had in mind when she began this endeavor. Clearly written and based on scientific evidence, this book serves as an introduction to MS and addresses the common questions that patients ask about this multifaceted disorder.

In sharing details of her own illness, Beth immediately forms a personal connection with her readers, whether they are patients afflicted with MS or their relatives or friends. One of the best recommendations that comes forth early in the text is that all patients need to search for physicians, nurses, and therapists who they can trust and who treat them with kindness and patience. Patients should feel secure and nurtured by the professionals who will be overseeing their health care. Beth then explains some basic definitions and terminology that neurologists use when discussing MS, such as optic neuritis, demyelination, brainstem lesions, etc. Many aspects of diagnostic testing and treatment options are often confusing for patients. Every reader will appreciate the author's honesty as she discusses some mildly invasive procedures that, to the patient, may not seem "mildy invasive" at all, such as the spinal taps and electrical tests that many MS patients need. There are also numerous alternative therapies about which there is limited scientific information. MS patients may wonder: Should I try acupuncture? Bee sting therapy? Chelation therapy? And everyone inquires about lifestyle changes: Is exercise safe with MS? Should I stop working? Does stress cause my attacks? Although these issues are not always clear-cut, the author tackles them and discusses their uncertainty.

From her personal struggles with MS and after extensive review of the established literature, Beth Hill has provided us with an inspirational, comprehensive manual, specifically written for patients. This book will serve as a resource to help many patients cope with their illness. It is clear that the author has a tremendous sense of responsibility and compassion for others who have this disorder. Her hard work will hopefully help others regain control of their lives and become informed participants in their health-care decisions. Most important, she has provided patients and families with hope so they can once again approach the future with optimism and pursue their dreams with the knowledge that a cure for MS is just around the corner.

—Joanne Wojcieszek, M.D., Neurologist
Director, Movement Disorders Program
Indiana University School of Medicine
Indianapolis, Indiana

Introduction

I never thought I would be writing a book on multiple sclerosis. And I certainly never thought I would develop the disease. I was young. I was healthy. I was superwoman! Or so I thought.

But life changes, and mine certainly did when I developed MS seven years ago. When I first heard those words, "You have multiple sclerosis," I felt lost. Immediately, mental pictures of people in wheelchairs flashed through my mind. I didn't know a great deal about the disease. So, like many other people with MS, I set out on a mission to educate myself.

I'll never forget the first book I picked up about multiple sclerosis. It was very technical. It explained all the theories on what MS is and how demyelination works. But at that time, I wasn't concerned with what MS is and what it could do to me. I already knew what it was doing. And I was scared. What I really wanted to know was "Why me?" and "What do I do now?" and "How do I cope with this?" The only books I could find that dealt with the "how" question concerned a lot of how-tos: how to choose a wheelchair, how to use a catheter. I remember looking through one of these how-to books and thinking, *Boy, this is going to get really bad!*

Multiple sclerosis can be devastating and more than a person can handle. A few months ago, I realized the necessity of having a book that tried to meet not only educational questions but also to offer a positive approach to management of the disease as well. I was reading an Associated Press article about Dr. Kevorkian, or Dr. Death. According to the article, twenty of the ninety-three people whose suicides he engineered had MS! I was immediately struck by multiple sclerosis's power to devastate people's lives. These gentle souls were so fatigued and tired of dealing with it every day that they no longer wanted to live—they wanted out.

I truly believe that people can sometimes have more than they can handle. Just like Dr. Kevorkian's patients, many of us can and do have more than we can handle. Life can be very difficult—sometimes unbearable. And MS greatly adds to that burden.

Out of these thoughts came the idea of *Multiple Sclerosis Q&A*. This book is designed to answer basic questions that you might have about MS and to offer guidance on what to do, who to contact, what to read, etc. The book is organized into three basic sections.

Part One is my story. I think reading anyone's story about MS is helpful. Not only does it help you know where other patients are coming from, but there are similarities in stories. Many people with MS experience the frustration of finally receiving a diagnosis. And even though there are a variety of MS symptoms, there are also many similarities from one patient to another. I think it helps to hear other people's stories and to know that they have the same problems you do.

For example, for many years now, I have had problems with my eyes. I see what I call "raindrops," which are blurry dots, as though someone has flicked water on your glasses. But of greater concern and frustration to me are the "lines" in my eyes. There are literally hundreds of stationary, hairlike lines crossing my line of vision in both eyes. I describe it as looking through a net. I once tried to explain the lines to an ophthalmologist. He didn't really understand and brushed them off as "floaters." However, when I read the story of another person with MS, she talked about "cobwebs" appearing in her eyes. This was exactly what I had! After reading her description, I knew I wasn't losing my mind. The lines were, in fact, a result of the MS. In the same way, I hope hearing my story will help you unravel some of the mysterious symptoms that you might experience with this strange, unpredictable disease.

Part Two consists of questions and answers, organized into eight chapters: "Defining Multiple Sclerosis," "History and Statistics," "Symptoms," "Diagnosis and Medical Tests," "Treatment," "Family Issues," "Lifestyle

Changes," and "Other Relevant Questions About Multiple Sclerosis." I tried to include questions that you might not see in any other books. I also tried to keep the answers short and simple.

Part Three of the book is what I call my Suggestions section. It includes information for people who have not yet been diagnosed but who think they have MS. "Twenty Things to Do if You Have MS" provides a helpful list of things that you should be doing after you are diagnosed. There are also pages with suggestions for friends and family members.

MS is a terrible disease, but there is good news. The good news is, a cure will be here soon! As a doctor once told me, if you have to have a chronic disease, MS is one of the better ones to have. MS is listed as one of the top diseases that experts believe will be cured in our lifetime. And now, with the use of one of the new disease-modifying drugs, you can significantly slow down the progression of the disease in your body. Scientists are also making progress on regenerating the myelin in rats—a significant development for all of us who have residual damage from attacks.

I hope that this book is helpful to you. Let's begin our journey together with my story.

PART I

. . . .

MY
STORY

. . . .

Everyone with MS has a story. From the onset of the first symptom, to the eventual diagnosis, to the ever-changing day-to-day struggles, it's usually not a simple story, and mine is no exception. Because this disease is so mysterious and so difficult to understand, I have found it extremely helpful to listen to the stories of others with MS. I have found similarities between their stories and mine. I have discovered that everyone suffers the same frustrations and fears when dealing with MS. I have also found incredible stories of strength and hope. There are so many wonderful, beautiful people out there with MS. By sharing our stories, we form a bond—a bond of friendship that allows us to continue on in our fight against MS. Rather than being one big "pity party," we find answers to questions, suggestions for adapting to and dealing with the disease, and strength. We receive encouragement from others who are in the same boat.

I've had MS for seven years now, although I have only had my diagnosis for three. It took me four years and ten doctors before I finally had an answer. From what I have read, this is pretty typical.

Before 1995, I was a very healthy, strong individual. I graduated from college with a master's degree in music and taught for five years as a music teacher. Then I went back to school and received another master's degree in communications. From 1990 to 1999, I worked in public relations as a writer for a Fortune 500 company in Atlanta. I loved my job. I worked long hours but still had time to exercise. In fact, some might have considered me an exercise fanatic. I exercised all the time. From the early eighties until my marriage and my first pregnancy in 1992, I exercised for two hours a day—walking, doing aerobics, lifting weights, swimming, and working out on a treadmill. Ridiculous, really, how much time I spent in the gym. Looking back now, I didn't really have a life. I went to work and then to exercise. In 1992, I became pregnant with my first child and went into premature labor. I was on bedrest for five months, which set my exercise routine back considerably. After my daughter was born, I began exercising again and got back into shape. In 1994, I became pregnant with my second child and again was put on bedrest. Up until September 1995, a few months after my second daughter was born, my health was very good. I was very strong and active and had lots of energy. But that would change quickly.

In 1995, I was living in Atlanta, Georgia, with my husband, Danny, and our two daughters when I began to notice that I was nodding off during the course of the day. I would fall asleep while talking, walking, or doing tasks. At the time, I thought, *Boy, I must be really tired to be falling asleep like this!* Finally I had one of these nodding-off experiences while driving on the freeway. If you have ever been in Atlanta and have driven on I-75, you know what an incredible experience it can be—five to six lanes of bumper-to-bumper traffic all going seventy-plus miles an hour. Not a great place to have a medical problem! In this case, the nodding-off episode lasted a little longer than usual, causing me to swerve in traffic. I made my way over to the berm, stopped, and sat for a while with my heart pounding and traffic whizzing by relentlessly. I realized at that moment that I needed to see a doctor for my exhaustion. How little did I know!

I made an appointment to see my primary-care physician. I told him that I was falling asleep during the day—falling asleep while at my computer, while walking, and even while driving. I told him about my I-75 incident and his eyes became large. He immediately set me up to see a neurologist. I saw the neurologist the following week, and he set me up for an EEG to test my brain-wave patterns. When the results came back from the test, he gave me some surprising news: "You're not falling asleep," he said. "You're having seizures. Small petit or absence seizures. As many as one hundred an hour." I sat there with Danny in shock. The neurologist's diagnosis was that I was epileptic, and he prescribed medication for the seizures.

Danny and I walked to the car in silence. Once we were inside, I turned to him and asked, "How can I be epileptic?" "You're not epileptic," my husband wisely answered. From our limited knowledge of seizures, we knew that they didn't just come on out of the blue. You were either born with them or you had a tumor or had been in an accident of some sort. None of those things applied to me. So we decided to seek a second neurologist's opinion before I went on any medication. By the time I saw the second neurologist a month later, the seizures had completely stopped. One month earlier, I had been having documented seizures. Now there were none. He had no explanation for the seizures, except to say that they might have been caused by stress or a hormonal imbalance due to the birth of my child.

I never really felt "well" after this time.

In May 1996 we moved to Grand Rapids, Michigan, and I started a small public relations firm out of our home. In September 1996, I woke up with a "weak" left leg. The leg almost felt as if I had had a partial epidural. I could walk on it, but I walked with a slight limp. I found it extremely difficult to climb stairs and could not step over a baby gate without lifting the leg with my hand. I went to our new primary-care physician in Grand Rapids. I will never forget that examination. He seemed very intent when examining my reflexes in that leg. He kept tapping and tapping the leg. And then he would stand back, stroking his chin, and stare at my leg. He did this over and over again. Then he stroked the bottom of my left foot with a little rubber hammer. He did this over and over again, too, and as he did, he'd murmur to himself, "Something's not right here. No sirree." I think perhaps he was the first to suspect something, although he didn't tell me what. He then sent me to a well-known neurologist in town, who did a lengthy examination. When he was finished, he told me to dress and wait in his office. When he came in, he had a tissue box, which he set before me and promptly said, "Are you going to need these now or later?"

"It depends on what you have to tell me," I replied. He then explained that I had neurological damage all over my body, not just in the leg (although more severely in the leg). "You either have a brain tumor or MS," he blatantly diagnosed. "We're going to do an MRI to see which it is." I left his office in shock, angered by his insensitivity and afraid for my future. By the time I actually had the MRI two weeks later, the problems with my leg had cleared up. To my surprise (and the doctor's), the MRI was normal. "I still think you have MS, and I want to do a spinal tap," he said when I saw him during my follow-up visit. At that point, my leg seemed fine and I wasn't all too impressed with that doctor! The whole incident had been one big pain in the patootee, so the last thing I wanted was a new pain in my back. I hoped that it was another freak event and opted out of the spinal tap and vowed never to see that doctor again.

Six months later, in February 1997, I went to a new family doctor, complaining of fatigue and muscular weakness. He sent me to a specialist in internal medicine, who then did yet another MRI, evoked response potential tests, an EEG, and the dreaded spinal tap. All tests were normal. He said he could find "nothing wrong" with me.

In March 1997, I again went back to that doctor, complaining of increased fatigue, numbness in my arms and legs, and muscular weakness. He talked with me and said that he couldn't really find anything. He said I didn't have MS but could possibly have a mixed connective tissue disease. I didn't feel at the time that he was really taking me seriously, so I decided that he would join my doctors-to-never-see-again list.

A few days later, I woke up with a completely limp left hand. I got in the shower and reached for the shampoo bottle, and it fell through my fingertips. I stood there with the water raining over my head and the tears flowing down my cheeks. Again and again, I tried to pick up the bottle and couldn't. It was then that I realized that this wasn't some freak event. It wasn't my imagination. It wasn't a bad dream.

Three days later, I once again returned to my primary-care physician. The numbness and lack of strength in my hand, which I now know was an MS episode, lasted exactly two weeks. I didn't want to go back to the internal medicine specialist, so he recommended that I take a trip to the Mayo Clinic.

Arranging a visit to the Mayo Clinic is no small matter. You have to arrange for all your medical records to be sent, not to mention making flight and hotel arrangements. Finally, in April 1997, I boarded a plane destined for Rochester, Minnesota. I spent a week there. Between visits to doctors and lab tests, I did research on what was wrong with me. At the time of my visit, I had very few symptoms. The numbness in my hand had cleared up. All that I had been experiencing at the time of my visit was a little numbness and tingling, and fatigue. All of my previous tests—MRIs, spinal tap, evoked response potential tests, and EEGs—had been normal. After a battery of tests and visits with a neurologist, she sent me to a psychiatrist. After spending less than an hour with me, he said I was suffering from postpartum depression from the birth of my second child a year earlier. "But I'm not depressed!" I answered angrily. "Yes, I know. And because of that I'm calling it an *atypical* postpartum depression." (Boy, if I wasn't depressed before that visit, I sure was afterward.)

The trip to Mayo was very discouraging for me. When I came home, I told Danny again (I had talked to him nightly by phone) what had happened and what the doctor's diagnosis was. I remember sitting on the bed with the unfilled prescription for an antidepressant in my hand. I still didn't feel I had received a correct diagnosis. "They're wrong, Danny," I said. "I don't have postpartum depression."

"Beth," my husband said gently, "they're the Mayo Clinic. They can't be wrong." But something told me they were. And now, because of hours of research at the Mayo Clinic, I had my own diagnosis for my suspected illness—multiple sclerosis. Though not yet diagnosed, I knew the cause. All of my symptoms pointed in that direction. Because of the problems I had had with doctors, I decided I would forget about getting help and just hope the symptoms would go away on their own. But MS doesn't work that way.

A year later, in the summer of 1998, I awoke one day and felt terrific. I was putting on my makeup, and I remember looking at myself in the mirror. *I feel good today,* I thought, as I put on my eyeliner. Then I stopped and looked directly into the mirror. *No, I don't feel good,* I thought. *I feel normal.* This was the first time in four years that I had felt normal. I discovered that I was pregnant a week later. I felt wonderful during the entire pregnancy—totally free of all previous symptoms, and not even fatigued! It was a joyous time.

In February 1999, I gave birth to my son. Everything went well, although I immediately began to feel fatigued again. I thought it was just the fatigue from sleep deprivation due to the nightly feedings. I hoped against hope that it wasn't the old monster returning. In the meantime, my home-operated public relations business was suffering. I specialized in crisis communications and often worked long hours during a crisis event. During one job, I flew to Tennessee and by the time I got there, I was so exhausted that I could barely walk through the terminal. After working just two hours talking to reporters, I told the client that I was ill and went back to my hotel. Although I worked the next day for fourteen hours, I began to realize that I couldn't continue at this pace. I began to question everything about my life. Even though I loved my work, it took me away from my children too much. I was a token mother at best. I began to seriously question whether the field of public relations was where I was intended to be.

Meanwhile, the monster continued its assault on my body. In August 1999, I burned my hand on the oven. I was making steak and, in my hurry, dropped the hot pad. I grabbed the metal rungs of the oven with my hand, and it didn't hurt. I could feel that it was hot, but not burning hot (even though the oven was set to "broil"). When I pulled my hand out, welts were forming where I had grabbed the rungs. I remember looking at the long welts and thinking, *You idiot. You've been hurt. Put your hand under the water.* This experience had a lightbulb effect on me. I realized then that I should have felt pain and that I had been hurt, but for some reason, my body couldn't feel it.

Also in August 1999, came another significant turning point in my life. My number-one client (who was wonderful) retired, but his replacement didn't seem as eager to use my services. Even though I had won numerous awards for their company, she seemed reluctant. In August, I took a trip to Atlanta to present a proposal to her. After only forty-five minutes, I realized that it was over and I thanked her for her time. Then, for the next six hours, I walked around Atlanta. I had just lost my largest client. It would take at least six clients to make up for all of the work that this client had given me. I knew that I didn't have the energy to both pursue new clients and to follow through with the work. It was over. My business was gone. The next day, I returned to Grand Rapids.

Two days later, I received a call from the Grand Rapids Public School system. I had applied as a teacher years before when we first moved to Grand Rapids, and they had found my application. They had an opening for a music teacher. The job would start the following Monday. Was I interested? I wasn't. I had burned out years ago as a music teacher. I had been unappreciated and mistreated by administrators. And yet I had loved my students. Was this my answer? Reluctantly, I again became a music teacher, in the Grand Rapids Public School system—a very poor intercity school district. I quickly found that I loved teaching. I loved my students, and, to my amazement, they seemed to love me.

Then in December, I went blind in an eye while teaching. *What now?* I thought. I finished out the day and again called my primary-care physician. He sent me to the hospital. After finding someone to watch our children, my husband joined me. I had another MRI, a blood test, and a CAT scan. And then, after the tests were completed, we waited. For more than five hours, not a single nurse or doctor came in to see me. Then finally, after midnight, a new physician walked in the door—the head of the ER. I looked at Danny and he looked at me. They were sending in the big guns; this wasn't going to be good. "We're sending you home." "What?" I practically yelled in surprise. "Did I have a weird migraine or something like that?" "No," he gently answered, taking my hand. "It looks like you have MS, Beth." I remember looking up at the ceiling light and thinking, *Bingo!* "Are you giving me a diagnosis?" I asked. "No," he said. "That's for the real experts to do. I'm sending you to see a fine neurologist. He is kind and very good at what he does. You'll be very happy with him."

A week later, Danny and I learned that he had been right. The new doctor was warm and caring—not the least bit ostentatious. I liked him immediately. But he didn't give me a diagnosis right away, either. He wanted to do one more test, another spinal tap. I refused at first. My first spinal tap had been very painful, and I didn't want a repeat performance. "We want to be one-hundred-percent sure that you have MS, Beth," he explained. He went on to explain that the medications for MS were not the kind of meds you can take "just in case." Each of them is administered by injection and can have side effects, not to mention that they cost more than $1,200 a month. "I want to be sure, and you need to be sure, too," he wisely advised me. So I reluctantly agreed to the spinal tap.

Although unpleasant, the second spinal tap was a breeze compared to the first. I went home and rested, wondering what the neurologist would tell me at my next appointment in two weeks. At 5:00 P.M., I received a call from his nurse. "The doctor would like to see you tomorrow at 8:00 A.M. And he would like for your husband to attend, too." Needless to say, I didn't sleep much that night!

The next morning, Danny and I were sitting in the waiting room when the doctor poked his head out and brought us back to his office. He sat down and we sat there, the three of us looking at one another in silence. I waited. I had waited a long time to hear it, and I didn't want to put the words in anyone's mouth. "Your spinal tap was abnormal," he said. Again, we sat in silence. Finally, he said, "You have MS, Beth." I sat back in my chair with a huge sense of relief.

My husband, on the other hand, was a little confused. "Do you mean that she possibly has MS?"

"No, it's definite. She definitely has MS," the doctor confirmed.

Finally! The moment I had waited for. After ten doctors, I finally had a diagnosis! We went home with materials from the Copaxone, Avonex, and Betaseron companies.

It's strange to say, but, after my diagnosis, I was elated! I was so relieved to finally know what was wrong with me, to know that I wasn't losing my mind, and to know that I could finally get help for my illness! To be able to fight back was so important to me. I've always been a fighter, and it's hard to fight something that you can't see. Now I knew what it was. It had a face and a name. I could fight.

I began my fight by choosing one of the medications used to fight MS. I joined the National Multiple Sclerosis Society and became involved locally. I also began an exercise program. And I continue to work as a music educator, although now only three days a week.

Things are not easy for me. I have my good days and my difficult days. In May 2000, I had my worst episode and used a cane for three months. I've been blind in my right eye six times now. These episodes last anywhere from three to six weeks. Although my sight has returned, I have some residual damage from these episodes. Halos have appeared around lights (such as car headlights, televisions, and lamps), making night driving virtually impossible for me, as well as the lines and blurry spots in my eyes that I mentioned earlier. These visual problems seem to be permanent. Besides the fatigue and the slight achiness I feel every day, the vision problems are probably the most frustrating, because I'm forced to look through the mess each day.

In general, my symptoms since 1995 have included:

- General overall fatigue (my greatest problem)
- General muscular weakness (difficulty climbing steps at times and fatiguing easily)
- Numbness and tingling in the hands and feet
- Growing stiffness and rigidity in my entire body

- Stabbing, shooting pains daily—usually in my hand or left foot (it feels like I have been hit with a little rubber hammer or shocked), but sometimes in my face
- General achiness, like having the flu
- Creepy-crawly feelings (like little ants) in my legs and arms, which become worse at night
- Inability to tolerate heat (I become extremely fatigued after a hot shower or bath and almost unable to function in the summer heat)
- Inability to feel pain in my left hand (the hand I burned on the oven)
- Inability to open jars or doorknobs with my left hand
- General feeling of shakiness, dizziness, and being unbalanced
- Changes in my gait (I now walk with a slight wobble)
- Noticeable changes in handwriting and difficulty in filling out forms (I should have been a doctor—I now have the handwriting to go with the profession!)
- Limp leg (three times)
- Limp hand (once)
- Problems with memory on occasions (as noticed by myself, Danny, my mother, and friends)
- Vision problems (blurriness, halos around lights, vertical lines, and gray spots)
- Petit seizures (twice)
- Tremors in both hands
- Depression, caused by fatigue

But even with all these problems, there is a good side to all of this. I appreciate life much more than I used to. I make a real effort to be a better mother and spend quality time with my children. I appreciate the generosity of my friends and the kindness of strangers. Even with the MS, my life is much better and much sweeter than ever before. Now, let's go to Part Two and answer your questions about multiple sclerosis.

PART II

Questions & Answers About Multiple Sclerosis

Defining Multiple Sclerosis

. . . .

What is multiple sclerosis?

An easier question might be: "What isn't multiple sclerosis?" MS displays a multitude of symptoms and can be very difficult to diagnose. To help make the definition a little easier to understand, I have divided it into four important points. Multiple sclerosis is:

- *A chronic disease.* A chronic disease is one that is not life-threatening, that won't just go away, and for which there is no cure (as of yet).
- *A disease of the nervous system.* Multiple sclerosis involves three areas of the central nervous system—the brain, the spinal cord, and the optic nerves.
- *A potentially debilitating disease.* This means that multiple sclerosis can sometimes cause disability in a patient.
- *Probably an autoimmune disease.* An autoimmune disease is one in which the body's immune system attacks itself. In the case of multiple sclerosis, the body attacks the myelin that protects nerves. Myelin is like insulation around an electrical wire—the wire being your nerves. MS destroys the myelin. When the myelin is gone, it is replaced with scars, or "sclerotic" tissue. With the myelin gone,

the messages can't be received. This often occurs in many places along your nervous system—hence the name *multiple sclerosis.*

What causes MS?

This is the key question in the study of multiple sclerosis. Scientists have narrowed causes of diseases down to the following eleven descriptive areas.

1. *Toxic.* Over the decades, numerous studies have been performed to study toxins in the environment. So far, all have been ruled out in the case of MS. (Examples of diseases in this category include emphysema. Emphysema, or chronic obstructive pulmonary disease, can be caused by the toxins found in cigarettes or cigars.)

2. *Vascular.* Many years ago, doctors thought MS was related to faulty blood circulation. Today, through advanced medical technology, we know that MS patients have the same vascular systems as the rest of the population. (Examples of diseases in this category include coronary artery disease and Raynaud's disease.)

3. *Metabolic.* Various theories about chemical imbalances in the body abound. Just search for multiple sclerosis on the Internet and you will see hundreds of listings for "guaranteed" cures related to a chemical or hormonal imbalance of some kind. The truth is that science has ruled out many nutritional and hormonal causes to date. There is no evidence, so far, that MS has a metabolic cause.

4. *Hereditary.* Recent studies have shown that there is a slight increase in MS in families. This could be because family members could be exposed to the same virus. Or it could be that children could inherit a genetic susceptibility to MS. A Canadian study of twins in 1986 found that 26 percent of identical twins had MS, while only 2.3 percent of fraternal twins both had the disease.

5. *Congenital.* A congenital disease is one that someone is born with. We are not born with MS; it occurs later. Most congenital theories have been ruled out as a cause of MS. (Examples of congenital diseases include cerebral palsy and cystic fibrosis.)

6. *Degenerative.* Degenerative diseases are diseases in which a part or parts of the body begins to die off due to an unknown cause (Alzheimer's disease is in this category). MS also used to be in this

category. Now, because MS is believed to be caused by an infection or an allergy, its placement has been moved. (Other examples of degenerative diseases include Parkinson's disease and amyotrophic lateral sclerosis [ALS].)

7. *Psychogenic.* A psychogenic disease is one that is brought about by an emotional stressor. MS is not thought to be psychogenic in nature, although some people believe that stress can be a factor in the course of the disease. (Post-traumatic stress disorder [PTSD] is an example of a psychogenic disease. For example, a woman who was sexually assaulted as a child may later develop tremors or seizures.)

8. *Tumors.* Tumors have never been suspected of causing MS. MS can sometimes be mistaken for a brain tumor, however, because they both cause patients to display some of the same symptoms.

9. *Trauma.* Like the psychogenic category, trauma is not considered to be a cause of MS. However, it is believed that trauma can bring about an attack.

10. *Infection.* For approximately one hundred years now, scientists have suspected that either a bacterial infection or a virus causes multiple sclerosis. At first, tuberculosis or syphilis was suspected, but both have now been ruled out as the cause of MS. Studies of spinal fluid in MS patients have shown high antibody titers (strengths) to the rubella virus (which causes measles), herpes simplex, Epstein-Barr, and others. A study in 1985 conducted at the Wistar Institute in Philadelphia implicated a retrovirus, human T-cell lymphotropic virus I (HTLV-I). In 1997, researchers at the National Institute of Neurological Disorders and Stroke in Maryland announced that their studies had shown a high incidence of HHV-6 antibodies in people with MS. Their research indicated that the herpesvirus, which causes the common childhood illness roseola, could be the culprit. The study of thirty-six people with MS found that two-thirds had HHV-6 antibodies. Other studies have indicated that chlamydia pneumoniae might be the cause. Most recently, researchers have discovered a possible link between the Epstein-Barr virus and MS.

11. *Allergy.* When you think of an allergy, you often think of someone who sneezes around cats or who might be allergic to dust or mold, or perhaps someone who has a life-threatening allergy to peanuts. These are all allergies to something in the environment.

What scientists believe happens with MS is that a person essentially becomes allergic to certain tissues in his or her own body. They believe that because of a problem with B-cells or T-cells, the patient's body begins producing antibodies that attack healthy tissue—in this case, myelin. This is called autoimmunity. (Examples of autoimmune diseases include rheumatoid arthritis, lupus, and myasthenia gravis.)

To summarize all this information: At the present time, the leading consensus about how a person develops multiple sclerosis is:

- that there is a slight genetic susceptibility to MS (not just one MS gene, but as many as twenty locations in the patient's DNA that may play a role)
- that MS is most likely caused by early exposure to a virus (with perhaps a twenty-year latency period)
- that there is a "trigger" of some sort that basically "turns the switch on"
- and that MS results from a problem in the immune system (possibly abnormal T-cell or B-cell production) in which the body's immune cells attack myelin

For example, a *possible* scenario of how a person develops multiple sclerosis might be the following:

- A person inherits a genetic predisposition to MS (heredity)
- The person contracts a virus as a child, perhaps chickenpox or measles, for example (infection)
- Approximately twenty years later, the individual is exposed to a trigger (perhaps the same virus)
- Then, because of a problem in the immune system with T-cells or B-cells (unknown at this time), the myelin is attacked (autoimmunity) and multiple sclerosis begins

It's easy to see how complicated multiple sclerosis is and how many factors must exist for you to develop the disease. I hope this better explains why it has been so difficult to find a cure for MS.

But can't some diseases have more than one cause?

Yes, many can. Cancer, for example, can be caused by exposure to chemical toxins, radiation, or viruses. It is also considered a genetic disease, because the information that determines what your cells do and how they grow are found in your genes. It is possible that MS has more than one cause, so it may end up being classified in more than one category—possibly genetic, infection, and allergy.

Why does MS occur?

There are volumes and volumes about this topic in medical journals—much more information than I could ever print here. The truth is that no one knows for sure why MS occurs and what goes wrong within the body. At the present time, it is believed that T-lymphocytes could be responsible. T-lymphocytes, or T-cells, are what the body uses to fight major disease. They are the "big guns"—the nuclear warheads of the body. For some reason, when a patient has MS, these T-lymphocytes attack the myelin as if it were an invader. During an MS exacerbation, abnormal levels of T-cells can be found in the spinal fluid of the patient. However, a new study by scientists at the University of California suggests that the culprit may actually be what are called B-cells, which produce antibodies. These antibodies attach to the myelin as it is being destroyed.

Currently, it is believed that MS is an autoimmune disease. Why the immune system attacks the myelin is still unknown. Whether the cause is T-cells or B-cells or something yet undiscovered, it is essential that researchers determine what causes MS. When we find the cause, the cure will be just around the corner.

Is MS similar to AIDS?

Except for the fact that they both involve the immune system, they have no similarities. Acquired immunodeficiency syndrome (AIDS) is caused by a virus—the human immunodeficiency virus (HIV). HIV is passed from person to person through bodily fluids such as blood or semen. Then, some people go on to develop AIDS. Others live a long life while being HIV positive.

There is no evidence to date that MS can be spread through human contact. There is *not* a multiple sclerosis virus like there is with AIDS (HIV). However, it is possible that faulty T-cell or B-cell production is triggered by a common virus, such as the childhood illness roseola.

Can I get MS from my spouse?

No. Currently, there is absolutely *no* scientific evidence that MS is spread from person to person. A study in 1995 concluded that MS clusters in families occurred because of shared genes, not because family members infected each other with multiple sclerosis.

What are the different categories of multiple sclerosis?

Experts have created four different categories of MS. Within each of these categories, the disease can be mild, moderate, or severe:

- *Relapsing-remitting multiple sclerosis (RRMS).* Approximately 70 to 75 percent of people with MS begin with a relapsing-remitting course. With RRMS, patients experience definite attack and recovery periods. These attacks can be twenty-four hours in length or last for a few months. Usually, patients fully recover, or they might experience some minor disability because of the attack.

  Before I was diagnosed and started one of the disease-modifying drugs, I had anywhere from four to twelve episodes a year. Some lasted a day or two, others lasted two weeks or more. One episode, my most severe, involved my left leg and hand and lasted three months. I now have some damage in my hand as a result of that episode. But since I started the disease-modifying medications three years ago, I have had only two episodes.

- *Secondary-progressive multiple sclerosis (SPMS).* Within ten years, 50 percent of MS patients who started with relapsing-remitting multiple sclerosis move on to develop secondary-progressive multiple sclerosis. With SPMS, the disease steadily worsens. There is a wide range of disability with SPMS. A patient's MS could worsen only slightly over many years, or it could worsen rapidly. Sometimes the disease can hit a plateau, during which it seems to maintain its current level of severity. With SPMS, the patient can also have occasional attacks.

  To summarize, secondary-progressive patients start out with relapsing-remitting, during which there are definite recovery periods, and then move on to experience a steady progression of the disease.

- *Primary-progressive multiple sclerosis (PPMS).* With primary-progressive MS, patients start out with a progressive course. PPMS patients do not experience definite attacks or recovery periods. PPMS can vary in rates of disease progression—from very mild to severe. Only 15 percent of people with MS begin with this course.

- *Progressive-relapsing multiple sclerosis (PRMS).* As with PPMS, the patient's symptoms continue constantly without remitting. However, with progressive-relapsing MS, the patient also experiences acute flare-ups (relapses). PRMS only occurs in 6 to 10 percent of those with MS.

What is "silent" MS?

Silent, or benign, MS is a form of MS that causes lesions but no neurological symptoms. Recent studies estimate that there is one person living with silent MS for every four people diagnosed.

What is an attack?

An "attack," or "relapse," of multiple sclerosis is the development of new symptoms or a significant increase of old symptoms. An attack must last twenty-four hours or more. New symptoms are an indication of inflammation and demyelination in the spinal cord or brain. The terms "exacerbation" and "flare-up" usually refer to a worsening of current symptoms. Many people use all four words interchangeably.

What causes an attack?

Researchers have not yet been able to determine what causes an episode. Many theories abound, including stress, infections, physical trauma, and even sudden weather changes. When scientists figure out exactly what causes an attack, we will be much closer to finding a cure.

Why do some attacks produce permanent damage but others don't?

When myelin is attacked, the surrounding area becomes inflamed. When the inflammation goes away, in most cases the myelin repairs itself. But if the attack is severe enough, or if the area has been repeatedly attacked, the myelin can be replaced by scar tissue, in which case the nerve signals are not received and damage is permanent.

Can stress cause an attack?

The verdict isn't yet in on this one. Many people with MS swear that it can. I know that the worst episode I ever had occurred after I broke up a fight at one of my schools. It was a potentially dangerous situation and had been extremely stressful for me. Two days later, I woke up with a limp leg and, after intravenous steroids, ended up using a cane for three months.

According to the book *Living with Multiple Sclerosis* by George Kraft and Marci Catanzaro, it isn't the moment of stress that causes an attack, but the attack seems to be an after-effect of the stressful situation. When we are under stress, our bodies produce high levels of adrenal corticoids, or adrenaline. After stressful events, our adrenaline levels drop rapidly, sometimes causing an attack. I believe this is what happened to me after

I broke up the fight. I didn't have an episode *during* the stressful event, but I had a major attack a few days later.

Can illness cause an attack?

Yes. Attacks often follow a bout of the flu. Influenza stimulates the immune system. Fever is also often a result of the flu. These factors, working together, can bring about a pseudo-exacerbation. If you get the flu or develop a high fever, it is important to keep your body temperature down. Taking a fever-reducing medicine such as acetaminophen as well as frequent room-temperature sponge baths is a must.

What is a "pseudo-exacerbation"?

A pseudo-exacerbation is the return or worsening of prior symptoms brought on by a high fever due to an infection. In these cases, symptoms subside after the infection is treated with antibiotics. For example, your vision might become blurry during the illness and then improve as you recover.

Can exercise cause an attack?

Research has indicated that exercise does not cause attacks. However, getting overheated during exercise can cause a temporary worsening of symptoms (such as blurred vision, fatigue, or weakness). Unfortunately, it is a vicious cycle. MS patients can become too tired to exercise, but if they don't exercise, their muscles will get weaker, and then every movement will take even greater effort.

From my research and my own personal experience, I believe exercise is one of the key elements (along with one of the medications) in fighting MS. You must fight the disease. You can't give in to it!

Can the nervous system repair itself after an attack?

To a certain extent, the nervous system can repair itself after an attack. However, even early relapses that appear to be minor can damage the actual nerve, not just the myelin. If the nerve cells are severed in two by a relapse, the damage is permanent and irreversible.

However, there is some very exciting and promising news for MS patients who have experienced what seems to be permanent neurological damage. Scientists have made major progress in their work on nervous system repair. A few studies include the following:

- Researchers led by Steven Goldman, M.D., Ph.D., at Cornell University Medical College have isolated immature oligodendrocytes in the brain that can mature into cells that produce myelin. Testing is continuing to determine the possibility of transplanting these laboratory-matured cells into people with MS.
- Goldman, along with other scientists, is also studying natural growth factors, which stimulate the brain to repair the damaged myelin.
- Dr. Jeffrey Kocsis of Yale University is studying transplanted myelin-making cells in rats. Results to date have been very promising.
- A Mayo Clinic scientist, Moses Rodriguez, M.D., has reported successful myelin repair in mice. This was achieved by injecting the mice with immune-system proteins called "monoclonal antibodies" (see page 58).
- Dr. Marie Filbin of Hunter College in New York is taking a different slant to the problem. She is studying why axons don't repair themselves. What she has discovered is that a component of myelin called MAG (myelin-associated glycoprotein) can actually keep axons from repairing themselves. Filbin is experimenting with natural growth factors called "neurotrophins" to see if they can block MAG and allow axons to regenerate.

As you can see, there is hope for those of us who have neurological damage from multiple sclerosis. Thanks to scientists such as these, and the work of the National Multiple Sclerosis Society, we could see some amazing developments in the next ten years with nervous system repair.

When I tell people that I have relapsing-remitting multiple sclerosis, they ask if I am in remission. I don't know how to answer. I'm not having an attack, but I sure don't feel like I'm in remission.

The name "relapsing-remitting" is somewhat deceptive. People with this type of MS have definite relapses or attacks, which then abate. However, very few people with MS are in total remission. Even between relapses, a person with MS can have severe fatigue, numbness, tingling, dizziness, visual difficulties, and a host of other symptoms.

How you answer this question depends on the relationship you have to the person asking the question and what you feel comfortable telling others. If the person is genuinely interested in finding out more about multiple sclerosis, you could explain in greater detail to them: "Most people with MS are never in remission. They have times when the MS is quiet, but they are rarely free of all symptoms." But in most cases, the following simple response works very well: "No. But I'm hanging in there. Thank you for asking."

HISTORY AND STATISTICS

. . . .

How long has MS been around?

We don't know for sure, but the earliest record we have is from the skeletal remains of a woman known as Lidwina van Schiedam. Lidwina lived in the Dutch town of Schiedam from 1380 to 1433. The "strange disease of the virgin Lidwina" is explained in detail in the excellent historical book *Multiple Sclerosis Through History and Human Life* by Richard Swiderski.

Who discovered MS?

It is difficult to know who really discovered MS. MS has been with us for a long time. We know, however, that physicians had some idea about MS as early as 1838. Autopsy drawings from that year show details of a disease that we now know as MS.

The person who is actually credited with discovering MS was Professor Jean-Martin Charcot, also known as the "father of neurology." He followed the course of one patient with MS, detailing the disease as it progressed. After her death, he performed an autopsy and discovered the characteristic MS plaques.

Who gets MS?

Scientists have helped us get a good picture of who gets MS. MS is:

- more common in Caucasians than people of African, Asian, or Hispanic backgrounds
- found two to three times more often in women than men
- more common in the higher socioeconomic groups (at least in the United States)

How many people have multiple sclerosis?

In the United States, approximately 350,000 people have received a diagnosis of MS. Numerous others are in the "probable" and "possible" categories. According to the National Multiple Sclerosis Society, a new case is diagnosed every hour.

At what age does someone usually develop symptoms of MS?

Most people are diagnosed with multiple sclerosis between the ages of fifteen and fifty, although there are cases of children younger than fifteen with the disease.

Is MS more common in certain parts of the world?

Yes, the disease is more prevalent in certain hemispheres. MS is:

- more common in northern parts of the northern hemisphere and southern parts of the southern hemisphere
- much less common in the tropics
- found in higher concentrations in locations between 40° and 60° latitude north

Does where you grew up make a difference in your susceptibility to MS?

Yes. As far as your chances for developing MS are concerned, where you grew up is more important than where you currently live, or at least a bigger predictor of your chances of getting MS. A person who was raised in the northern United States but has moved to the South has a greater chance of acquiring MS than someone who was raised in Atlanta, for example, and moved to Michigan.

Is MS an inherited disease?

MS is generally not considered a genetically inherited disease, but MS does occur more often within families. It is believed that people do not inherit the disease, but some people can inherit a genetic predisposition to MS. For example, a mother with multiple sclerosis will not automatically pass MS on to her children, but her children could inherit a genetic predisposition to the disease. In the United States, the average person without a parent with MS has about 1 chance in 1,000 of developing MS, while relatives of a person with MS have a 1 in 100 chance.

Having said that, for the person with a genetic predisposition to MS to develop the disease, there must be some triggering event to actually cause the disease. For example, a person doesn't inherit alcoholism from his parents. However, he might inherit a genetic predisposition to the disease.

Studies of identical twins have been helpful in this area. With both identical and fraternal twins, it is possible for only one twin to develop MS. However, there is a higher likelihood of both identical twins developing MS than both fraternal twins. There is also a higher likelihood of the second identical twin developing "silent," or benign, MS.

Is there an MS gene?

No. Research has shown that as many as twenty locations in the human DNA may play a part in MS susceptibility. No single gene is responsible—

it's much more complicated than that. Scientists believe that someone with MS must inherit a certain *combination* of several genes to develop the disease. It is also believed that, since the immune system is involved with the myelin damage in MS, at least one of the susceptibility genes will involve the immune system. (In 1991, the NMMS began working with an MS gene bank at the University of California. The project's goal is to search for susceptibility genes in MS patients. If you are interested in being a part of this project, please call the NMMS at 1-800-FIGHT-MS and select option 1 to ask to speak with your chapter's research advocate.)

SYMPTOMS

· ·

What are the symptoms of MS?

When you look at the list below, you'll see one of the reasons why MS is so difficult to diagnose. Everyone's symptoms are different and could include any combination of those listed. MS can also mimic a variety of other illnesses and diseases.

In brief, possible symptoms of MS include (I will go into greater detail on some of these symptoms in subsequent questions):

- Blurred or double vision
- Loss of vision in one eye
- Pain when moving one eye
- Moving or "jumping" field of vision
- Appearance of numerous or new "floaters" in one or both eyes
- Dysesthesias, or altered sensations, such as itching, burning, or a feeling of "pins and needles"
- Electrical shock sensations in the neck and spine
- Paresthesias or pain (could also include trigeminal neuralgia or facial pain)
- Numbness and tingling
- Weakness in an arm or leg

- Feeling "heavy"
- Loss of strength anywhere in the body
- Development of a limp or dragging a foot
- Fatigue
- Dizziness or vertigo
- Poor balance or staggering
- Tremors
- Headaches
- Seizures
- Cognitive impairment (thinking and memory problems and confusion)
- Depression
- Changes in handwriting (due to lack of control and sensation in the fingers and hands)
- Tightness around the chest (also called the "girdle sensation")
- Paralysis
- Spasticity (involuntary muscle stiffness and sudden movements or spasms)
- Slurred speech
- Bladder or bowel problems (including urgency, incontinence, and control problems)
- Sexual difficulties
- Babinski reflex (a neurological indication of MS in which the big toe moves up rather than down when the side of the foot is stroked)

(Note: These symptoms can also be indicative of other problems. Check with your doctor if you experience any of them.)

What kind of vision problems could I possibly develop with MS?

People with MS can develop numerous problems with their eyes. Some experience diplopia (double vision). Others have nystagmus (jerky eye movements). Both of these conditions often improve after an attack. Optic neuritis is another common visual problem. In the case of optic neuritis, the demyelination occurs in the optic nerve, and the patient may experience blurred vision, color blindness, blind spots, and pain when the eye is moved. Often, one of the very first signs of MS is optic neuritis.

I was recently diagnosed as having optic neuritis by my ophthalmologist. Does this mean that I will develop MS?

Not necessarily. According to *Inside MS,* the magazine of the National Multiple Sclerosis Society, 50 to 70 percent of people who have optic neuritis will develop MS within two to fifteen years. This means that 30 to 50 percent of people diagnosed with optic neuritis do not develop MS. Of those who develop MS, optic neuritis rarely leads to total blindness.

You mentioned altered sensations in the list of possible symptoms. What kind of altered sensations are you talking about?

Dysesthesias, or altered sensations, can include the following:

- Feelings of hot or cold or wetness when there is not a source of the sensation
- Tearing or ripping pain
- Unpleasant feelings such as "pins and needles" or electric shock sensations (often in the face and neck) or creepy-crawly feelings (like little ants on or under the skin)
- The "girdle sensation," which feels like you have a tight band constricting your chest area
- Brief, intense itching called paroxysmal itching

I have experienced many of these sensations from time to time. In one instance, I had the feeling that there was something wet and hot on my backside. Of course, nothing was there. This sensation continued for three days. I also often experience creepy-crawly feelings in my body at night. It feels like little ants are crawling deep inside my body.

Dysesthesias is a *neurologic* disorder. It is not an allergy, and it is not psychosomatic in nature. Corticosteroid lotions will not help these conditions. Note: Paroxysmal itching can be relieved by taking medication such as hydroxyzine or an over-the-counter antihistamine.

Do people with MS experience pain?

According to a survey conducted by Dr. Yuan Bo Peng at the University of Texas, 55 percent of the people studied experience what is called "clinically significant pain" at some point during the course of the disease. Almost half (48 percent) experience chronic pain.

Types of pain can include:

- Trigeminal neuralgia (stabbing pains in the face)
- Lhermitte's sign (an electric-shock sensation brought on by flexing the chin toward the chest)
- Dysesthesias, or altered sensations, that can cause pain as well as discomfort
- Muscle spasms, tightness, and aching (spasticity)

There are numerous treatments available to help MS patients experiencing pain, including:

- Medications such as gabapentin, oxcarbazepine, diphenylhydantoin, carbamazepine, amitriptyline, and over-the-counter drugs such as Tylenol, Advil, and Motrin
- Anti-inflammatory drugs such as baclofen, tizanidine, or ibuprofen, which can be taken for spasticity
- Heat, physical therapy, and massage are also very helpful
- Exercise to help manage stiffness and pain; stretching exercises can be a proactive way to help stay pain-free
- Alternative therapies, including yoga, meditation, acupuncture, and hypnosis
- In severe cases of trigeminal neuralgia (stabbing pains in the face), a surgical procedure called "rhizotomy" is sometimes recommended

There are many options available to those of us with MS who suffer from pain. For additional information, contact the Trigeminal Neuralgia

Association at (609) 361-6250 or www.tna-support.org and the American Chronic Pain Association at (916) 632-0922 or www.theacpa.org.

What is spasticity?

Spasticity usually involves the legs, but can also occur in the arms. Spasticity can include both sudden muscle jerking or contractions and stiffness.
Treatments often include:

- medications such as the antispasticity drugs baclofen, tizanidine, and diazepam
- daily stretching exercises

What is tremor?

Tremor is rhythmic shaking movement in the muscles, which you can't control. The most common type of MS-related tremor is caused by loss of myelin on nerve fibers in the cerebellum (part of the lower back section of the brain), specifically the part called the "thalamus," which controls voluntary muscle movement and balance.

One of the first MS symptoms I developed was a tremor in my right hand. The tremor and fatigue have been the two MS symptoms that have been with me from the beginning. The tremor in my right hand makes writing difficult (my handwriting is almost illegible now), and it is sometimes noticeable to others. I find that it gets worse when I am tired or overheated.

Possible treatments for tremors include:

- Medication, including clonazepam, isoniazid, and evodpa
- Physical and occupational therapy
- Neurosurgery
- Electrode implants

What is vertigo?

Dizziness is a very common symptom of those suffering from MS. Much less common is the spinning sensation known as vertigo. When people think of "vertigo," they often think of the Alfred Hitchcock mystery starring Jimmy Stewart. In the movie, Stewart suffers from vertigo because of a traumatic experience. Unlike Stewart's character, MS patients suffer from dizziness and vertigo that are neurologic in origin and are caused by damaged areas in the brain.

Symptoms of dizziness and vertigo often respond well to anti–motion-sickness drugs such as meclizine, scopolamine, ondansetron, promethazine, or baclofen and diazepam.

(Please note: Dizziness can also be caused by other disorders such as ear infections and tumors. See your doctor if you experience any of these symptoms.)

What about fatigue? Is fatigue a common symptom of MS?

Fatigue is the *most* common symptom. According to the National MS Society, fatigue occurs in 80 percent of people with MS. People with MS often say their fatigue is unlike anything they have ever felt. I describe it to my friends as feeling like having mononucleosis. An "I want to lie down on the floor" kind of tired.

In my younger, pre-MS days, I used to fantasize about handsome movie stars. Now I fantasize about where the best place to sleep would be: a hammock under a shady tree, under a quilt on a winter afternoon, under a beach umbrella on the beach . . . The fatigue never leaves me. To me, this is the largest problem and causes me the most grief. The most difficult thing for me is not to be able to join in on a fun activity because I am too fatigued and need to rest. I sometimes feel that I am wasting my life away sleeping.

The severe fatigue associated with MS appears to be unique to the disease and is related to myelin damage. In some cases, the fatigue can be disabling.

What kind of cognitive impairment problems can MS produce?

Because multiple sclerosis often occurs in the brain, it can affect many parts of your thinking, memory, and emotions. In most cases, these problems are minor and a slight annoyance. I'll give you a few examples of times when I have experienced these kinds of problems.

Many years ago, before I was diagnosed and when I still had my public relations business, I was doing work for a client in Atlanta. Having lived in Atlanta for many years, I was very familiar with the city and outlying areas. After finishing the job for the client, I called a good friend and asked if I could pay her a visit. I began driving to her house, a place I had visited hundreds of times before, and realized that I couldn't remember how to get there! Not only could I not remember, I couldn't even remember the names of streets and highways. It was as if the entire map of Atlanta had been wiped from my memory!

Another incident occurred recently while I was at my school. I was walking down the hallway when a young lad asked me, "How much is five times seven?" I began to answer him and then realized suddenly that I couldn't remember. Not only could I not remember what five times seven was, I couldn't remember any of my multiplication tables! I called my doctor's office and asked what to do. "Get out your flash cards and relearn them," the nurse told me. So I purchased flash cards and relearned the multiplication tables. I'm still a bit shaky on a few of the higher numbers, but most of the information is back.

I relate these memory problems to computer problems. It's as if you're clicking on a computer file and, when it opens, it's empty. You know the information was there, but now it's gone.

Besides directions and math, these problems can include difficulty recalling a particular word to finish your sentence, recalling names, recognizing faces, remembering important dates such as anniversaries and birthdays, and various types of confusion. I often have conversations with my mother in which she will say, "I told you that. Don't you remember, dear?" And no, I certainly don't.

To combat the damage MS is doing to your brain, you need to keep your mind active. Go to school, learn something new, read, do puzzles and word games, anything to keep your mind fresh. If you are losing brain cells, grow a few new ones! In addition, there are medications that can help with cognitive difficulties. Your neurologist can also refer you to a therapist who can pinpoint the areas of damage and help you learn how to work around these issues. Whenever I go anywhere now, I carry a map, and the address and phone number of the person I am seeing. I also use a planner for my daily tasks. When I complete a task, I cross it off.

Can MS cause depression?

Yes. With MS, the depression can be brought on by the constant fatigue of the disease, or it might be of biological origin. Demyelination in certain parts of the brain can change your moods and actually cause depression. So, if you are depressed, it might be a natural reactive consequence of the disease, or it could be a biological or organic result of the demyelination. Regardless, antidepressants and counseling can be of great benefit. I have been on an antidepressant for a year now, and I believe it has been very helpful. My mother calls them my "sweet" pills because they make me more even-tempered. Wouldn't it be nice if the whole world could take a sweet pill?

Please note: Depression can be a side effect of using Avonex, Betaseron, or Rebif. If you experience depression while taking any of these medications, contact your physician.

What kind of bladder dysfunction can MS cause?

MS-related lesions can cause numerous types of urinary tract problems. Lesions in the brain and spinal cord can disrupt the transmission of signals between the organs of the urinary system and the brain.

According to the National Multiple Sclerosis Society, types of bladder dysfunction in multiple sclerosis include: urgency (inability to delay urination), frequency (the need to urinate in spite of having voided very recently), nocturia (the need to urinate during the night), incontinence (the inability to control the time and place of urination), dribbling (uncontrolled leakage of urine), and hesitancy (delay in ability to initiate urination even though the need to void is felt).

There are numerous medications for treating bladder dysfunction. Propantheline bromide, imipramine, and oxybutynin relieve bladder spasms. Tolterodine reduces contractions of the muscles surrounding the bladder. Desmopressin (a nasal spray) reduces the amount of urine in the kidneys.

Other treatments include drinking plenty of liquids (including cranberry juice to guard against urinary tract infections) and medical aids such as catheters to remove urine.

What kind of bowel problems can MS cause?

Constipation is a very common problem for people with MS. Physical inactivity, limiting the amount of liquids due to bladder problems, and some medications used to treat MS can all contribute to constipation. In addition, damage to the brain and spinal cord caused by MS-related lesions can disrupt the signals indicating the need for a bowel movement.

Proactive treatments for constipation include drinking more fluids, exercise, and the use of bulk supplements such as Metamucil, Perdiem, FiberCon, Fiberall, and Citrucel and stool softeners such as Surfak and Colace.

What kind of sexual problems can MS cause?

Multiple sclerosis can cause numerous problems with both sexual performance and intimacy. The severe fatigue associated with MS can cause a disinterest in sex. Depression and anxiety can also limit libido. Embarrassment and fear about leaking urine or having an accident during intimate moments can cause partners to stop having sex.

Of course, intimacy and sexual performance are two different things. Intimacy is a feeling of attraction, gentleness, and love. It is a sharing between two people. Intimacy can include kissing, massage, hugs, sharing thoughts, talking, and laughter. For the purpose of this question, we will deal with the sexual performance problems associated with MS.

For women, sexual performance problems include a lack of sensation, disinterest in sex, uncomfortable or painful sensations, vaginal dryness, and difficulty reaching orgasm. Treatment for sexual problems in women include using medications (such as phenutoin and carbamazepine to decrease sensory discomfort), the use of lubrication ointments, and Kegel exercises to strengthen vaginal muscles.

For men, sexual performance problems include difficulty achieving or maintaining an erection, lack of sensation, disinterest in sex, premature ejaculation, and inability to ejaculate. Medications for treating sexual problems in men include medications such as Viagra and Alprostadil.

There is an important point about all of this: Don't be afraid or embarrassed to tell your neurologist about any difficulties you might be having in this area. This is a very common problem with those who have MS, and I guarantee that your doctor has heard it before! There are many different things that can be done to help you, including medication and therapy. Just don't be afraid to discuss it. Also, please be aware that some drugs used to treat depression may also reduce libido or lead to difficulty reaching orgasm. The good news is that the problem can often be remedied by taking drugs like Viagra, Wellbutrin, or amantadine in addition to your antidepressant. Ask your doctor for more information.

Finally, one of the best methods of dealing with intimacy and sexual performance issues is to talk about them with your partner. Keeping the lines of communication open between partners is essential for a healthy and happy relationship.

Can an MS symptom last for just a short period of time?

Yes. Called "paroxysmal symptoms," these episodes can last a few seconds or a few hours. Sometimes they recur repeatedly during the day. Symptoms can include muscle cramps, pain, tingling, difficulty initiating movement, visual problems, and altered sensations.

My first paroxysmal symptom occurred before I was diagnosed. I was Christmas shopping at a large mall, when suddenly I couldn't walk. I couldn't move my legs! I stood there in the middle of the aisle, with people passing me on both sides. I didn't know what to do! Out of embarrassment, I didn't reach out to anyone. What would I have said—"Excuse me, but for some reason I can't walk"? So I stood there and tried to act nonchalant. I looked around as though I were gazing at holiday decorations. Finally, I was able to shuffle my feet a little, so I would shuffle and then stop and look at decorations, shuffle, and stop again—just to look normal. Finally, I shuffled my way to a chair and literally fell into it. After about an hour, I felt the feeling come back, and I was able to hobble my way out of the mall.

Another incident occurred every day for a two-week period and lasted for only thirty minutes each time. Each morning, when I would awaken, my right eye would not open. The first time it happened, I literally panicked, running around and asking my husband if my eyeball was still in my head. When I realized that, yes, it hadn't rolled away during the night, I felt much better about it. It got to be a real challenge, especially putting on makeup with one eye closed. I looked like Popeye, minus the pipe and spinach.

What course will my disease take?

It is very difficult to tell how multiple sclerosis will progress for you. MS displays a totally different set of symptoms for each person. One person might have a milder version of the disease and then one day wake up unable to walk. Still another could have one severe episode and then go into complete remission and never experience another episode. One thing that sets MS apart from other diseases is its unpredictability!

Having said that, there are some guidelines that are used to help predict prognosis. According to the National MS Society, people who experience the following tend to have a milder course of the disease:

- Long intervals between attacks
- Complete recovery from attacks
- Attacks that are sensory in nature (such as numbness and tingling)

People whose early symptoms include tremor or trouble walking, or who have frequent attacks with incomplete recoveries, tend to follow a more progressive course.

Can MS "burn out"?

Yes. In some cases, a person with MS will have relapses for a few years and then go into total remission, never to have another episode.

Will I end up in a wheelchair?

According to a survey completed *before* the new disease-modifying drugs became available, 25 percent of those with MS ended up needing a wheelchair or being totally incapacitated. It is possible, with the availability of the new medications, that the general public's association of MS with wheelchairs may soon be a thing of the past.

Can MS be cured?

Not yet, but it can be slowed down through the use of one of the disease-modifying drugs, which will be discussed later in the "Treatment" section. At the present time, there are four from which to choose: Avonex, Betaseron, Copaxone, and Rebif.

When do experts believe a cure will be found?

It is difficult to say, although many experts believe that a cure will be found in our lifetime—perhaps even in the next ten years. Scientists have made tremendous progress, however, with the development of the disease-modifying agents Avonex, Betaseron, Copaxone, and Rebif. These drugs significantly slow down the progression of the disease. It is possible that very soon we may be able to nearly halt the progression of the disease altogether! Although not a cure, it is the next best thing until a cure for MS is found.

DIAGNOSIS AND
MEDICAL TESTS

. . . .

How is a person diagnosed with MS?

Very carefully! At the present time, magnetic resonance imaging (more commonly referred to as an MRI) is generally used as the main tool for diagnosing MS. Having said that, however, there are no medical tests that can *absolutely* rule out MS. Generally, a physician needs to be a detective of sorts to determine that MS is the culprit behind your symptoms. Sometimes a decision can be made within a few weeks, but often it takes years to get a definite diagnosis. It's estimated that the average MS patient sees eight doctors before finally receiving the correct diagnosis!

Before the development of the MRI, it was much more difficult to diagnose MS. It usually took years of observation before the patient finally received a definite multiple sclerosis diagnosis. Today it is easier to receive a definite diagnosis of MS because of the MRI. We still have categories of MS, however, because even a positive MRI is not a conclusive test for MS. Other diseases can cause lesions that show up on MRIs, so a neurologist must consider other factors in making his or her diagnosis. Also, a patient can have a normal MRI and still have MS.

The categories are as follows:

- *Possible MS* means that the diagnostic tests are inconclusive but that MS cannot yet be ruled out (for example, a patient might have tingling in the fingers and weakness but a normal MRI and spinal tap).
- *Probable MS* means that a patient could have definite attacks with recovery but negative lab tests or he or she might have attacks in the same spot (for example, a patient with a limp leg and normal tests or another patient with abnormalities in just one area on an MRI).
- To receive a diagnosis of *Definite MS,* a patient must have experienced two attacks with at least one month between the attacks. There also needs to be more than one area of damage to the central nervous system as indicated on an MRI.

Can MS be mistaken for other illnesses or vice versa?

Yes. Other medical problems that can cause symptoms similar to those of MS include:

- Strokes
- Vitamin B deficiency
- Diabetes
- Pinched nerves
- Infections
- Tumors
- Lupus
- Arthritis
- Acute disseminated encephalomyelitis (ADEM)
- Sjögren's syndrome
- Binswanger's disease
- Amyotrophic lateral sclerosis (ALS)
- Mixed connective tissue disease
- Chronic fatigue syndrome (CFS)
- Lyme disease

(For more information about this topic, please see "Disorders That Mimic Multiple Sclerosis" in NARCOMS' Fall 2002 issue of *Multiple Sclerosis Quarterly Report*.)

My doctor just told me that I have MS. I think I've had it for years! How did he arrive at this decision now?

If you aren't sure how he arrived at the diagnosis, by all means ask! There is, however, a basic rule of thumb for diagnosing MS:

1. A patient must have experienced two attacks. These attacks must be separated by at least one month.
2. There needs to be more than one area of damage to the myelin in the central nervous system (either in the brain or the spinal cord). (Note: Perhaps the reason I was not diagnosed immediately was because early MRIs were done on my spinal cord. In the early stage of the disease, my MS seemed to settle primarily in the right side of my brain.)

What are the medical tests that are used to pinpoint MS?

Numerous tests are used to help make a diagnosis of MS, including:

- *Medical history.* This involves reviewing your list of symptoms and how long each lasted. (Even after you have been diagnosed, it is a good idea to keep a running list of all attacks. This includes a description of the symptom, the start and end dates of the attack, which doctor or doctors you saw, what tests you had done and where, and any other information you believe could be helpful.)
- *Neurological examination.* During the examination, the physician will test your reflexes and muscle strength, as well as your ability to feel pain, temperature, touch, and vibration. The physician will test your vision. He may also do numerous coordination and bal-

ance tests. After the examination, the physician will usually recommend one or more of the following tests.

- *Magnetic resonance imaging (MRI) scan.* An MRI is often the first step after a neurological examination. It's a noninvasive test that uses a magnetic field and radio waves to scan the body and produce computerized images of body tissues. Doctors will examine these images and look for signs of MS, which often show up as small spots in the spinal cord and brain.

- *Spinal tap, or lumbar puncture.* During this procedure, doctors use a needle to remove spinal fluid. Then they look at the concentration of immune cells in your spinal fluid, as well as looking for the presence of oligoclonal bands. Found in the spinal fluid of about 90 to 95 percent of people with MS, these oligoclonal bands indicate increased activity in the patient's immune system. (Once the oligoclonal bands are positive, they will remain positive for the rest of the MS patient's life.)

- *Evoked potential tests.* During this test, doctors use electrodes to record how quickly your brain picks up messages. There are three types: visual, auditory, and pain-stimulus tests.

- *Blood tests.* These are often done to rule out other causes for your symptoms. At this time, there are no blood tests that can detect MS.

The following questions discuss these tests in greater detail.

What can I expect during an MRI?

If you have ever seen a photograph of an MRI scanner, it looks like something from outer space. The patient is put on a small bed that is glided into a cylinder-shaped scanner. The procedure is not painful and is usually not invasive. (Sometimes the patient is also given a small injection of a "contrasting material," which allows doctors to better see areas in the nervous system.) Depending on which part or parts of your body are being scanned, the procedure can take a few minutes or more than an hour. Unfortunately, the scanner is very loud! You may be given earplugs, but even with the plugs, you will hear loud knocking and buzzing sounds. The sounds are not frightening, and usually the technician will describe them to you before your MRI begins. Some facilities do not use earplugs and will allow you to listen to music during your MRI. The tube can also make some people feel claustrophobic. To alleviate this problem, some hospitals now have "open MRIs," which are better tolerated by patients with claustrophobia.

The first time I had an MRI, they did a scan of my entire spinal column, which seemed to take forever. This particular MRI had small, fun stickers in the visual area of the cylinder, which helped give me something to focus on. The important thing to remember is that you are not trapped. The technician can pull you out anytime you wish.

I've had an MRI, but nothing showed up that was abnormal. Does this mean I don't have MS?

Not necessarily. When doctors first started using MRIs to help diagnose MS, it was often believed that a negative MRI meant the patient didn't have MS. Now research has shown that lesions can be so small that even an MRI can't pick them up. And in the beginning stages of the disease, MRIs are often negative. You can have a negative MRI today and then have the MS make its appearance just a few months later.

According to the National Multiple Sclerosis Society, "A normal MRI does not absolutely rule out a diagnosis of MS. About 5 percent of patients who are confirmed to have MS on the basis of other criteria do not show any lesions in the brain on MRI. These people may have lesions in the spinal cord or may have lesions which cannot be detected by MRI."

Spinal taps can also be normal, even if a person has multiple sclerosis. If the test is done while the disease is inactive (or in a remitting phase), there may be no evidence of acute inflammation. However, if someone has had oligoclonal bands detected in the past, this indicator of chronic inflammation will always remain positive for the duration of the disease. (In other words, if you have an abnormal spinal tap with evidence of inflammation, subsequent tests will also be abnormal.)

My neurologist once explained this to me. He said that by the time anything is showing up on the tests, you almost don't need any tests to identify the disease—it has already become obvious when the patient experiences a limp hand or blindness in an eye, for example. I know this was certainly true in my case! For the first four years, the MS didn't show up on any tests I had been given. Numerous MRIs, a spinal tap, and evoked response potential tests were all normal. Then one day, every test showed abnormalities.

What can I expect during a spinal tap?

I'll be honest here: Spinal taps aren't fun. But when done by a knowledgeable, experienced professional, they should only be mildly uncomfortable. A spinal tap takes about fifteen minutes from start to finish. Before the procedure, a physician will numb the area in much the same way a dentist does, by injecting a small amount of anesthetic into the lower part of your back. (If the procedure is done correctly, this should be the only brief pain you will have.) After the area is numb, the doctor will insert a thin, hollow needle into your spine to remove a small amount of cerebrospinal fluid. Often, X-ray equipment is used to help the physician guide the needle. Then the doctor will slowly withdraw a small amount of cerebrospinal fluid. During this time, you will feel some pressure and you may feel slightly uncomfortable. When they have extracted some fluid, the needle is removed. For a brief second, your body will jerk slightly. (This is normal and will not hurt you, like the reflex your knee has when tested in a doctor's office.) After the procedure, a small bandage is applied to the injection site. Patients are usually told to rest for the remainder of the day. This is done to allow the opening to heal and to reduce the leakage of cerebrospinal fluid. (Doctors also request that someone drive you home after the test.)

I have had two spinal taps. During the first spinal tap, the doctor didn't use the X-ray equipment, and the pain was excruciating. The second time around, the X-ray equipment was used, and it felt only slightly uncomfortable. I highly recommend the X-ray equipment! (If your neurologist requests a spinal tap, ask if equipment is used to help guide the needle. If not, request that the procedure be performed at a hospital that has this technique available. You might have to travel to another hospital in another city, but it will be worth it!)

Also, there is a small chance that you could get a whopper of a headache after the spinal tap. I had that experience. Sometimes, they need to do another procedure, called a "blood patch," to clear up the headache. I had one of these. Basically, they take a small amount of blood from your arm and insert it into the area where you received the spinal tap.

Although I would have preferred not to have a spinal tap, it was necessary in my case to receive the diagnosis. And then, having received the diagnosis, I could get help for my disease. Although it was unpleasant, I have never regretted having had this procedure done.

What can I expect during an evoked response test?

During an evoked response test, harmless electrodes are attached to the patient's head. These electrodes connect the patient to an electroencephalograph (EEG), a machine that records the patient's brain waves.

There are three different kinds of evoked response tests: visual, auditory, and sensory.

During the most common visual test, the pattern-shift visual evoked response (PSVER), a checkerboard pattern is flashed in front of the patient's eyes while the patient sits in a chair. Computers record the amount of time it takes for the brain to receive the impulse. Slow transmissions indicate abnormalities of the optic nerve.

The auditory test is called the brain stem auditory evoked response (BAER). This test records the amount of time it takes the signal associated with a ten-second click to reach the brain. This particular test can indicate a brainstem lesion. According to Louis J. Rosner and Shelley Ross, the authors of *Multiple Sclerosis: New Hope and Practical Advice for People with MS and Their Families,* 46 percent of MS patients have abnormal BAER tests. However, hearing difficulty is seldom a serious problem for people with MS.

The final test is the somatosensory evoked potential (SSEP). This test can determine spinal cord and brain stem lesions measuring electrical currents. During this test, electrodes are attached to your scalp, and small amounts of electricity are delivered to your body via the finger, wrist, or knee. Computers then measure how long it takes for the messages to be received in your brain. Unfortunately, this test can be a little bit painful, because you are receiving mild electrical shocks.

Are there any new tests being developed to help diagnose MS?

Yes. A new medical instrument that might help solve some of the brain's mysteries is the whole-head magnetoencephalography sensor system (or MEG). Similar to the MRI, the MEG measures the tiny magnetic fields produced by the neurons in the brain. The MEG looks like a helmet and could help reduce the cost of such instruments from $3 million to less than $500,000.

TREATMENT

. . . .

How can I find a good neurologist?

There are numerous ways to find a good neurologist. To be quite honest, often it is a trial-and-error approach. However, you can speed up the process by using the following guidelines:

- Find a primary-care physician whom you trust and ask which neurologists he or she recommends.
- Although the National Multiple Sclerosis Society cannot recommend particular neurologists, they do have a list of NMSS-affiliated neurologists and clinics (see the appendix).
- Talk to other people who have MS. Ask them which neurologists they have seen and who they like the most. Ask them who they are seeing now. Ask them which neurologists to avoid.

It is very important that you find a neurologist who is kind and knowledgeable. You are going to have a long relationship with this doctor. It should be a good one. If you aren't satisfied, keep looking.

Which drugs are used to fight MS?

The MS disease-modifying drugs are Avonex, Betaseron, Copaxone, and Rebif. All four drugs significantly reduce the frequency and severity of MS attacks, delay the onset of disability, and reduce the amount of injury to the brain as indicated on MRIs. The chart on pages 52–53 might briefly answer any questions you have about the four drugs.

In 1998, the National Multiple Sclerosis Society issued its first statement recommending the use of one of these disease-modifying agents as early as possible for relapsing-remitting multiple sclerosis.

Can someone take one of these medications if they have "probable" MS?

As of February 2003, you can. For many years, the U.S. Food and Drug Administration (FDA) did not allow any of the disease-modifying medications to be used by those not yet diagnosed with multiple sclerosis. There were numerous reasons for this restriction at the time. First, the medications were, and still are, extremely expensive. In 2003, they cost more than $14,000 a year. Second, taking these medications doesn't entail just popping a pill. All four medications are given by injection— although the four manufacturers (Biogen, Inc.; Berlex Laboratories; Teva Marion Partners; and Serono International) are currently doing research on oral versions. Finally, the medications are not without side effects. Avonex, Betaseron, and Rebif can sometimes cause liver damage, and users must be monitored with blood tests every few months. They can also cause depression and suicidal thoughts. All four drugs cause pain and inflammation at the injection site.

However, in February 2003, the FDA extended the labeling of Avonex to include individuals who have experienced one clinical episode and who have an MRI scan showing evidence of the characteristic MS plaques. This is a *very* important development. Because MS is such a difficult disease to diagnose, it can sometimes take years for a patient to receive a definitive diagnosis. By that time, substantial damage to the central nervous system can occur.

THE MS DISEASE-MODIFYING DRUGS
(Interferons and Copolymers)

	AVONEX	BETASERON	
Chemical name:	Interferon beta 1-a	Interferon beta 1-b (or copolymer-1)	
Marketed by:	Biogen, Inc.	Berlex Laboratories	
How it works:	Immune-modulating drug	Immune-modulating drug	
How you take it:	Intramuscular injection	Subcutaneous injection	
Dosing frequency:	Once per week	Every other day	
Needle size:	1¼" length	½" length	
Storage:	Refrigerated	Room temperature	
Side effects:	Flulike symptoms, depression	Flulike symptoms, depression	
Approximate cost:	$1,200 a month	$1,200 a month	
Necessary monitoring:	Liver function and blood count	Liver function and blood count	
Indication:	Reduces frequency of relapses	Reduces frequency of relapses	
Support programs (available to NMSS members and nonmembers):	MS ActiveSource 1-800-456-2255	MS Pathways 1-800-788-1467	
Websites for more information:	www.avonex.com	www.mspathways.com www.betaseron.com	

COPAXONE	REBIF
Glatiramer acetate	Interferon beta 1-a
Teva Marion Partners	Serono International
Synthetic protein that serves as a myelin decoy	Immune-modulating drug
Subcutaneous injection	Subcutaneous injection
Every day	Every other day
½" length	½" length
Refrigerated	Refrigerated
Injection site reactions	Flulike symptoms, depression
$1,200 a month	$1,200 a month
None	Liver function and blood count
Reduces frequency of relapses	Reduces frequency of relapses
Shared Solutions 1-800-887-8100	MS LifeLines 1-877-44-REBIF
www.copaxone.com www.mswatch.com	www.rebif.com

For example, it took me four years to receive a positive diagnosis. In that time, I had more than twenty episodes. By the time I was diagnosed, I already had some permanent damage, including blurred vision and blind spots, as well as losing a substantial amount of strength in my left hand.

Things are changing very quickly in the treatment of multiple sclerosis. Hopefully, by the time this book is in print, the other disease-modifying medications—Copaxone, Rebif, and Betaseron—will also be available to those with probable MS.

Which of the disease-modifying medications should I choose?

The choice you make depends on which one you prefer and the recommendation of your physician. If you have definite MS, it is imperative that you choose one of the disease-modifying drugs and start taking it as soon as possible. Your future depends on it!

My insurance doesn't cover any of the disease-modifying medications! What should I do?

This is a problem. In the United States, only half of people with MS are using one of the disease-modifying medications.

For many years, Medicare did not pay for any of the disease-modulating drugs. As of August 2002, however, Medicare now covers Avonex because it is administered via intramuscular injection. The injection must be done in a doctor's office. The National MS Society is currently advocating for Medicare's approval of the other three disease-modifying drugs.

If your insurance does not cover any of the disease-modifying medications, you and your physician are your best advocates. Don't assume that you're out of luck. All four of the drug companies have service representatives to help people in your situation. They will work with you to find options. You might even be able to participate in a study! Don't give up until you have called everyone and checked out your options. For more information, call a service representative at the following numbers:

- MS ActiveSource (Avonex) at 1-800-456-2255
- MS Pathways (Betaseron) at 1-800-788-1467
- Shared Solutions (Copaxone) at 1-800-887-8100
- MS LifeLines (Rebif) at 1-877-44-REBIF

For more information about insurance and paying for the disease-modifying drugs, please see the following articles:

- A wonderful article about health-care advocacy was written by Dorothy Northrop, director of clinical programs at the National Multiple Sclerosis Society, titled "Getting Disease-Modifying Drugs in the U.S." (*InsideMS,* Summer 2002)
- "Lower-cost Prescription Drugs" by Seana O'Callaghan gives summaries about the various resources for prescription drug assistance. (*InsideMS,* Winter 2002)

And don't forget that the National Multiple Sclerosis Society is also your advocate! Call your local chapter about any problems you are having with access to the disease-modifying medications.

Are oral versions of these drugs available?

It's not as simple as it might seem. Many drugs become inactivated when they make their journey through the digestive tract, but scientists are conducting numerous studies in the hopes of finding a way around this hitch. These include the following:

- Phylogenzym, a combination of three enzymes that modify immune-system activity, has been going through testing in Europe since 1994.
- Three oral versions of Betaseron are currently in phase II development.
- Biogen, Inc. is also doing safety studies on an oral version.
- Oral versions of interferon, interferon alpha and interferon tau, are also being investigated.
- The oral drug valacyclovir (Valtrex) is being tested at one U.S. site. This drug is used to fight the herpesvirus. The study is based

on the hypothesis that MS is in part caused by the human herpesvirus 6.

- Another study, based on the fact that many women go into remission during pregnancy, uses an oral version of the pregnancy hormone estriol. The researchers of this U.S. pilot study are following twelve women with MS during a two-year time period and will gather information on relapses and disability.

As you can see, there is a great deal of research going on in this area!

What about combining medications?

This seems like an excellent idea, doesn't it? And the experts are already ahead of you. Several clinical trials are already under way, including the following:

- A trial in Europe, which will test the use of both Avonex and the immune-suppressing drug azathioprine (Imuran)
- Another European trial in which patients receive intravenous mitoxantrone (Novantrone) and steroid methylprednisolone for six months, followed by two years of Betaseron
- In 1999, a small trial began in the United States to test the effectiveness of both Copaxone and Avonex on thirty-two people with relapsing-remitting MS
- Another small trial being held at three U.S. medical centers to determine the safety of a single intravenous dose of Antegren (a monoclonal antibody that blocks immune cells to the brain) followed by weekly doses of Avonex

What about Novantrone?

The drug Novantrone (mitoxantrone) was released by Immunex Corporation (now Amgen) in 2001. It has been approved for use on secondary-progressive, progressive-relapsing, and (worsening) relapsing-remitting MS. It is not indicated for primary-progressive MS. (See the "Defining Multiple Sclerosis" section for more information on the categories of MS.)

Novantrone is given once every three months by a short five- to fifteen-minute IV infusion. In a two-year study, patients taking Novantrone had no worsening of their disability, significantly fewer relapses, increased time to first treated relapse, and significantly fewer new lesions. On the downside, Novantrone can have serious side effects. Patients treated with Novantrone can develop heart problems and must have regular testing. In addition, because of the risk of injury to the heart, there is a limit on the total lifetime doses a patient can receive, approximately eight to twelve doses in two to three years.

For more information on this drug, call 1-800-5NOVANTRONE, or log on to www.novantrone.com.

Can someone with progressive MS take Avonex, Betaseron, Copaxone, or Rebif?

Not yet in the United States, but probably very soon. Early results from a study by Biogen, the manufacturer of Avonex, claim that double the standard dose of Avonex significantly slows the progression of disability in people with secondary-progressive MS. The data analysis is still ongoing for this study. The National MS Society believes the data will be used to petition the FDA to approve the use of Avonex for those with secondary-progressive MS.

In Europe, Canada, and Australia, Betaseron has been approved for treatment of secondary-progressive multiple sclerosis.

Approximately 50 percent of people with relapsing-remitting multiple sclerosis advance into the secondary-progressive form within ten years. Many members of the MS community believe it is absolutely essential that these medications are approved in the United States to help those with secondary-progressive multiple sclerosis.

Is there anything else that is being done for people with secondary-progressive MS?

Yes. There are numerous large studies currently in progress that could affect current therapies for secondary-progressive MS. These include:

- A large trial that is testing IV gamma globulin in Europe and Canada. Gamma globulin is another immune-modulating treatment. It is made from immune antibodies from blood donors. Results should be available this year.
- A T-cell vaccination trial cosponsored by the National Multiple Sclerosis Society and the National Institutes of Health. In this treatment, T-cells are removed, deactivated, and reinjected into the patient. Scientists hope that the T-cell vaccination will neutralize the body's attack against myelin.
- Possible treatment for secondary-progressive MS using the cancer treatment Taxol. A new trial in Canada will test a reformulated version of this drug on 189 people with secondary-progressive MS. Scientists speculate that this immune-suppressing drug might allow the myelin to repair itself.

Are there any new medications on the horizon?

Yes. One drug is the monoclonal antibody natalizumab (Antegren). Preliminary studies on the drug Antegren have shown a significant reduction in the number of patients experiencing relapses. Delivered by intravenous infusion, Antegren is designed to stop damaging immune cells from going into the brain and spinal cord. Antegren works by attaching to a protein found on white blood cells. Preliminary studies on the drug have shown a significant reduction in the number of patients experiencing relapses. Elan Corporation (Dublin, Ireland) and Biogen, Inc. are currently working on the development of Antegren. Further testing will be required before the drug can be approved.

Another drug is Lipitor, an oral drug that is used to lower cholesterol. A current study by scientists at the University of California has shown that Lipitor has the ability to modify and inhibit certain immune responses in mice. Clinical trials will be necessary before it can be determined that the drug can help those with MS.

Which medications are used for major attacks?

For acute attacks, most physicians prescribe intravenous corticosteroid medications such as methylprednisolone (Solu–Medrol) for three to five days. Other commonly used corticosteroids include dexamethasone, prednisone, betametasone, and prednisolone. Some physicians also prescribe oral prednisone for minor attacks.

Corticosteroids are used because they help close the damaged blood-brain barrier as well as reducing inflammation in the nervous system. They will reduce the duration of the attack but will not influence the subsequent course of the disease.

Are there any side effects from being treated with corticosteroids?

Many people report few side effects except for slight bloating and moodiness. However, short-term use of corticosteroids can cause any of the following side effects:

- increased appetite
- indigestion
- nervousness
- difficulty sleeping
- headache
- increased perspiration
- growth of facial hair
- decreased or blurred vision
- water retention
- lower resistance to infection
- changes in blood sugar levels of diabetic patients
- possible birth defects if used during pregnancy
- mood changes (from mild to severe)
- long-term use of corticosteroids can cause cataracts, osteoporosis, and weight gain

What other medications are used to treat the symptoms of MS?

There are many! Here are just a few of the more common medications:

OTHER DRUGS USED TO TREAT MS SYMPTOMS

SYMPTOM	WHAT IT IS	
Spasticity	muscle spasms and stiffness	
Tremor	involuntary shaking	
Constipation	difficult bowel movements	
Trigeminal neuralgia	facial pain	
Paroxysmal itching	unexplained, severe itching	
Vertigo	spinning sensation	
Fatigue	severe tiredness	
Bladder dysfunction	urgency, frequency, nocturia, incontinence, dribbling, hesitancy	
Paresthesias	pain	
Depression	feelings of sadness and helplessness	
Erectile dysfunction	difficulty achieving or maintaining an erection	

*Please note that the SSRI drugs may cause sexual dysfunction.

BRAND-NAME DRUGS USED TO TREAT IT	GENERIC DRUGS USED TO TREAT IT
Baclofen, Zanaflex, Dantrium, Valium	lioresal, dantrolene, diazepam, tizanidine
Inderal, Mysoline, Klonopin, Symmetrel, Sinemet, Isoniazid	propranolol, primidone, clonazepam, amantadine, levodopa
Dulcolax, Colace, Sani-Supp suppository, Metamucil, Lactulose	bisacodyl, docusate, glycerin, psyllium hydrophilic mucilloid
Dilantin, Tegretol, Neurontin, Trileptal	phenytoin, carbamazepine, gabapentin, oxcarbazepine
Atarax	hydroxyzine
Valium, Phenergan, Meclizine, Dramamine	diazepam, promethazine
Symmetrel, Cylert, Provigil	amantadine, modafinil, pemoline
Detrol, Pro-Banthine, Tofranil, Ditropan, DDAVP nasal spray	imipramine, oxybutynin, propantheline bromide, tolterodine, desmopressin
Tegretol, Elavil, Amitril, Neurontin, Trileptal, Pamelor, Dilantin	amitriptyline, gabapentin, nortriptyline, phenytoin, carbamazepine
Selective Seratonin Reuptake Inhibitors (SSRIs)*: Paxil, Zoloft, Prozac, Celexa, Lexapro. Tricyclics: Elavil, Pamelor, Tofranil, Sinequan. Others: Remeron, Effexor, Valium	fluoxetine, paroxetine, sertraline, venlafaxine
Prostin VR, MUSE, Viagra	alprostadil, papaverine, sildenafil

What kinds of therapies are available to MS patients?

There are many kinds of therapies available to you, including the following:

- *Physical therapy (PT).* Physical therapists help you work to increase strength, flexibility, and balance. Their services could also include explaining the proper use of canes, walkers, and wheelchairs.
- *Occupational therapy (OT).* Occupational therapists help patients find the best ways to alter their environments to reduce fatigue. This could include techniques and exercises as well as adaptive devices for the home, car, and office.
- *Speech therapy.* Speech therapists work with MS patients who have trouble speaking or swallowing.
- *Cognitive rehabilitation.* Specialists in cognitive rehabilitation help patients find ways to improve and compensate for mental functioning problems, such as memory loss, attention deficit, and information processing.
- *Psychological counseling.* Mental health professionals—such as counselors, psychiatrists, psychologists, and social workers—help individuals with MS and their families deal with the pressure of having the disease. Counseling sessions can include many topics such as relationships, changing roles in the family, depression, employment concerns, and numerous other issues.
- *Sex therapy.* Sex therapists help couples deal with communication, intimacy, and sexual performance problems.

There are so many illegitimate claims of curing MS. What about alternative practices?

According to the Federal Trade Commission, there are literally hundreds of websites promoting phony cures for multiple sclerosis, so you have to be very careful when surfing the Internet for medical information.

It's easy to be fooled. Ellen Burstein MacFarlane was one of these people. In 1986, she was working as an investigative consumer reporter for WCPX-TV in Orlando, Florida. She also had MS. In her article on the National Multiple Sclerosis website, "Please Be Careful," she explains how she was duped by a physician with incredible credentials who claimed his program could cure MS. After paying him $100,000 for treatment, her condition deteriorated. She now uses a wheelchair and must have twenty-four-hour nursing care.

So what exactly is an alternative therapy? According to George Kraft and Marci Catanzaro's *Living with Multiple Sclerosis,* any treatment "that has not been proven to work in standard clinical trials may be called alternative." This doesn't necessarily mean that some alternative therapies are not effective or that your doctor wouldn't approve of your using them.

So how should you decide if you should use an alternative therapy? In Virginia Foster's article, "Clear Thinking about Alternative Therapies," she gives the following guidelines:

• Discuss the alternative therapy with your doctor before using it
• Find out if the alternative practitioner works with conventional doctors
• Talk to people who have used the treatment
• Investigate the background of any treatment provider
• Determine the costs
• Proceed with caution
• Do not abandon your conventional therapy
• Document your experience
• Keep your doctor up to date on any other treatments you would like to try

What are some alternative therapies for MS?

The answer to this question could fill another book! (For more information on alternative therapies, read *Alternative Medicine and Multiple Sclerosis* by Allen C. Bowling.) There are many wonderful alternative therapies, such as massage, tai chi, and yoga. These kinds of alternative therapies promote overall emotional, physical, and spiritual well-being. And yet, for every positive therapy, there are at least ten alternative therapies that are useless, expensive, and even harmful. These therapies are often marketed as cures for MS. Honestly, there is no cure for MS yet, and anyone who claims to be able to cure it isn't being truthful. Experts who have spent most of their lives studying the disease haven't solved the puzzle yet. It is a complicated disease, so finding the cure isn't going to be simple, either.

Below I have given just a small list of alternative therapies and recommendations on their usage. The recommendations are not my own but are given after months of research and discussions with experts on their opinions.

ALTERNATIVE THERAPIES FOR MS		
ALTERNATIVE THERAPY	**WHAT IT IS**	**EVALUATION**
Acupuncture	Ancient Chinese method of treatment in which fine needles are inserted in various parts of the body	May be useful in treating pain associated with MS
Chiropractic therapy	Physical manipulation of parts of the body	Helps relieve back pain
Massage therapy	Rubbing or kneading of parts of the body to aid circulation	Useful for relief of pain and spasticity and relaxes the muscles
Tai chi	Ancient Chinese system of meditative exercise	Lowers stress, promotes relaxation, relieves fatigue, improves balance
Bee sting therapy	The use of bee stings several times a day	Painful, dangerous (due to possible anaphylaxis or allergic shock), no value
Hyperbaric oxygen	Chamber is used to deliver high concentrations of oxygen	No value, expensive
Reflexology	Areas of the feet represent various parts of the body. The appropriate area of the foot is then massaged.	Assumptions of this therapy appear questionable. However, therapy is noninvasive and inexpensive

ALTERNATIVE THERAPY	WHAT IT IS	EVALUATION
Yoga	Meditation and exercise technique	Benefits include improved flexibility, relaxation, and increased muscle strength
Replacement of dental fillings	Removal and replacement of silver and mercury amalgam fillings	Ineffective and expensive
Aromatherapy	Use of scented oils through massage, inhalation, or hot baths	Helps with relaxation (note: hot baths can aggravate MS symptoms)
Chelation therapy	Intravenous injections of crystalline acid to remove heavy metals from the bloodstream	Ineffective, dangerous, can cause kidney damage, could be fatal

Will a special diet help my MS?

It would be nice to believe that a special diet of some sort could cure MS—if we eat this or don't eat that, we will be magically cured. There are many websites promoting one diet or another for MS patients. The truth is that there is no scientific evidence that any special diet cures MS. Controlled studies exploring the relationship of MS and diet have shown that your diet has little effect on the course of the disease.

Having said that, good nutrition is important for good health. A diet that is low in fat and high in fiber is essential. Both the American Heart Association and the American Cancer Society have recommendations on what constitutes a healthy diet. Also, keeping your weight down can help you battle the fatigue and mobility issues associated with MS. This, of course, is true of everyone, not just those with MS. Consult your doctor before starting any diet plan.

Will vitamins and minerals help my MS?

The truth is most people don't follow a healthy, well-balanced diet all of the time. Some of us *never* follow a healthy diet. Just drive down any major street and count the number of fast-food restaurants! Every day we eat too much junk, too much fat, and too many chemicals.

Having said this, most of us need a multivitamin of some sort to help us fill in the gaps in our eating habits. Your physician or a *registered* dietitian can recommend a good multivitamin for daily use. (Make sure your dietitian is registered. Many people who call themselves dietitians are really not dietitians. Your doctor or local chapter of the National Multiple Sclerosis Society can give you a list of registered dietitians in your area.) Consult your doctor before taking any supplements.

What are megavitamins? Will they help my MS?

Treating MS with megavitamins is based on the hypothesis that MS is caused by a vitamin deficiency. Studies have shown no correlation between vitamin deficiency and MS. While vitamins are essential for good health, megavitamins can actually be harmful. Too much of vitamins A, B_6, and D can cause nerve and liver damage. In addition, too much of one vitamin can sometimes cause a deficiency in another. Consult your doctor before taking any supplements.

Will medicinal herbs help my MS?

Herbs work like drugs in that they can bring about changes in bodily functions. They can be both helpful and harmful. Please note that some herbal supplements should not be taken in conjunction with certain prescription drugs, because they can affect the drugs' effectiveness. For example, Saint-John's-wort should not be taken along with a prescription antidepressant drug.

The following herbs have relevance to those with MS. The first three may be beneficial for many with MS; the last three, while having attractive benefits, could actually exacerbate MS symptoms.

MEDICINAL HERBS*

NAME OF HERB	WHERE IT COMES FROM	RECOMMENDATION
Ginkgo biloba	An antioxidant that comes from a tree native to China	Recommended: Helps decrease immune-cell activity, can inhibit blood clotting
St.-John's-wort	Made from a yellow flower	Recommended: Used as an anti-depressant but should not be used along with other antidepressants, could interact with other drugs including Elavil, Pamelor, Tegretol, Dilatin, and Mysoline
Cranberry	A fruit grown in North America	Recommended: Used to treat urinary tract infections
Valerian	Made from a root of a flower	Not Recommended: Used as a sleep aid, could increase the sedating effects of prescription medicines
Asian ginseng	An herb used by Chinese for centuries	Not Recommended: Claims to enhance physical performance, could stimulate the immune system
Echinacea	Made from a flowering plant	Not Recommended: Used to treat the common cold, could stimulate the immune system

*Always check with your doctor before starting a new herbal medication.

Do amalgam dental fillings cause MS? Will having the fillings removed make my MS go away?

No and no. Studies have shown that having amalgam fillings removed does not cause any changes in multiple sclerosis symptoms. Besides, cases of multiple sclerosis have been documented since the 1400s, long before amalgam fillings even existed.

FAMILY ISSUES

. . . .

We would like to have children.
   Is this still a possibility?

Generally, physicians do not discourage couples from having a child. Research has shown that pregnancy does not have a worsening effect on MS symptoms. In fact, MS often goes into remission during the course of the pregnancy. Issues to consider before having a child include:

- Reasons why you and your partner would like to have a child
- Your age and the level of disability you currently have because of your MS
- Your support system, including spouse, friends, and family
- Work issues, including time allowed off and insurance issues

How does pregnancy affect MS?

The majority of studies conducted on pregnancy and MS have shown that most women with MS do very well during pregnancy. Some women even seem to go into remission. However, the chance of an attack increases by 50 percent during the first three- to six-month post-partum period. Many women also report having their first attack right after the birth of a child.

When I was pregnant with my third child, I knew I was pregnant before I even used a pregnancy test. As I was getting ready for work one morning, I looked into the mirror and thought, *I feel good today.* Suddenly, I realized that I didn't feel good—I felt great. And then it dawned on me: I felt normal. It was then that I realized I was pregnant. I hadn't felt normal in a long time. It was great. Unfortunately, three months after the pregnancy, the MS returned with another relapse.

I have never regretted having my children. Sometimes it gets difficult, especially when I get extremely fatigued. But the benefits far outweigh the difficulties I experience.

Can any of the disease-modifying drugs be used during pregnancy?

At this time, Avonex, Betaseron, Copaxone, and Rebif have *not* been approved for use during pregnancy. Therefore, a woman must decide either to start a family and delay treatment or go on one of the disease-modulating drugs.

Right before I have a period, my MS symptoms worsen. Is there a correlation?

Studies so far have indicated that there may be a slight increase in MS symptoms during menstruation. Hormonal shifts as well as changes in core body temperature could explain the changes in MS symptoms during your period.

Will I give MS to my child?

You cannot give multiple sclerosis to your children. There is a slight chance, however, that you can pass on a genetic predisposition to MS to your offspring. The odds of your child actually developing MS are small—between 1 and 5 percent. Many people (including myself) believe that experiencing the love of a child is far more important than this small percentage.

According to the National Multiple Sclerosis Society brochure, "Pregnancy," the risk of a child developing MS is as follows:

- If no one in the family has MS: 1 in 1,000
- If mother has MS and the baby is a girl: 1 in 50
- If father has MS and the baby is a boy: 1 in 100
- If a sibling has MS: 1 in 20 to 50
- If a fraternal twin has MS: risk is the same as other siblings
- If an identical twin has MS: 1 in 3

In addition, this question may not even be relative by the time your child reaches maturity. Hopefully, we will have a cure by that time and the question will be moot.

Can family counseling help?

When I say that I have MS, my husband (only halfway kidding) says, "No, the whole family has MS!" And he's right. When one person has MS, the whole family is affected—the spouse, children, grandparents, neighbors, and friends. In our family, our week has to revolve around my MS. Every other day, I must take a nap or I can't function the following day. I can't do any heavy lifting and I must have assistance opening jars or taking heavy dishes out of the cabinets. Depending on my fatigue level, time must be allotted for me to rest. Driving at night is also a problem. When I go out with friends for a "girls' night out," someone else always has to drive. Even the neighbors help by carrying my groceries into the house or cleaning when I have an attack.

For many people, these kinds of changes can cause major upheavals in their lives and the lives of their families. Counselors can often help you find creative and positive solutions to these changes. Your local chapter of the National MS Society can also be helpful in this area by recommending programs, support groups, and counselors.

For some people, the idea of going to a counselor is embarrassing;

they believe that there is a stigma attached to seeing a counselor and that it is a sign of some sort of failure. This is not true. Going to a counselor can be a sign of strength—that you recognize there is a problem and you want to find positive ways to resolve it. This is a good thing! If you are still embarrassed, remember that no one needs to know except you, your family, and your counselor.

One additional note: For counseling to work, you and the counselor need to be a good fit. Sometimes you might need to try a few on for size before you find someone with whom you feel comfortable. Keep trying until you do. Don't give up!

What's the best way to tell children about MS?

The general consensus of experts today is that children, even young children, should be told when someone they know has MS. The explanation should be given in a nonemotional, age-appropriate way.

When I was diagnosed with MS, my two oldest children were four and six years old. My husband and I sat them down and explained that I had a disease called multiple sclerosis ("MS" will be easier for young children to remember). We told them that sometimes I might be a little tired or that maybe my legs wouldn't work very well. The children were wide-eyed when I said I would be giving myself a shot (or "poky," as we called them) daily. They thought that was pretty exciting and were interested to see if Mommy could really do it! We also assured them that I was not going to die and would always be there to take care of them.

At the school where I teach music, I didn't tell my students until I had my first noticeable attack. The older students were very interested about the disease and asked numerous questions. One teacher even used the illness as a research project in the library! The younger children seemed to take it fairly well, too, until one little five-year-old burst into tears at the sight of my cane. "Are you going to die?" he whimpered. I was startled and said, "No, I'm not going to die. But look what I can do with this cane!" Then I turned the cane around and used it like a hook to pull him to me and give him a hug. After that, all the little ones would come up to me and ask, "Mrs. Hill, can you hug me with your cane?"

I've noticed that my having MS has helped my young children in many ways. They seem more accepting of people with disabilities. They are very willing to help when I have an attack. (My second child even offered to let me borrow her teddy bear for a while!) They even seem a little braver during medical procedures, such as shots, because their Mommy gets one every day. It is difficult to tell yet how it will affect them as adults, but I hope that they will learn how to face adversity with strength and optimism.

How do I help my children cope with my disease?

Children are much more resilient than we know. Sometimes people with MS believe that their illness will have devastating effects on their children. Often, it is the opposite that occurs.

When we shelter children from life's disappointments and hardships, we do them a disfavor. Living with adversity can teach children strength, tolerance, fortitude, kindness, and the ability to handle change.

There are numerous things you can do to help your children cope in a positive way with your MS, including the following:

- Be a strong role model. When you have an episode, tell them that "this too will pass."
- Explain to them how they can help you. Give them opportunities to be helpful. Praise their efforts.
- Explain the illness to them in a gentle, nonthreatening way. Always answer their questions.
- Don't hide your illness from your children. Children often pick up on nonverbal cues and will know something is wrong.
- Spend quality time with your children. Ideas include reading a good book, watching movies, and painting together, or taking them to see a play or a basketball game. There might be some things that you can't do with your children, but that doesn't mean you can't be a good parent.
- Use humor whenever possible. Laughter can lighten our burdens.
- Children can fight MS, too, by participating in the MS Walk. If you can't walk or ride beside them, perhaps your spouse or one of your friends can!

- Printed materials are available from the National Multiple Sclerosis Society for your children. These include *Teen InsideMS* magazine and *Keep S'myelin,* a fun newsletter for five- to twelve-year-olds.
- Sometimes children benefit from individual or family counseling. Don't be afraid to get this kind of help for your child.

Are there any other suggestions that you have for coping with multiple sclerosis?

Yes. I believe that spirituality and reflection of any kind help many people. My own personal faith in God helps me during the down times. Even with the MS, my life is much better and much sweeter than ever before. God has been there to guide me—not to cure me, but to help me find strength and help when I need it. Likewise, you may find some kind of meditation or spiritual reflection helpful as you and your family react to the disease.

Belonging to a religious community has also been helpful for me. When I had a severe episode and was on bedrest for weeks, members of my church took turns bringing meals for my family. It's reassuring to know that there is a group of people out there who pray for me and care about my well-being. I'm grateful for them.

LIFESTYLE CHANGES

. . . .

Does heat make the symptoms of MS worse?

Temporarily, yes. When your body temperature rises, nerve conduction slows down. This can cause someone with MS to feel like a wet noodle. Many people with MS complain about feeling miserable in the summer and not being able to venture outside. Air-conditioning is really essential for someone with MS. In some cases, it can even be tax-deductible as a medical expense. Cooling vests—vests specially designed to hold ice or gel packs around your torso—are also helpful.

I love taking hot bubble baths! Can I still do this?

This is really up to you. Taking a hot bath can make you feel weak, but not everyone with MS is affected by heat. You need to determine how much heat affects you and alter your activities as such.

What about saunas or hot tubs?

Hot tubs and saunas are really out. Unlike a bath, which cools rapidly, hot tubs and saunas are made to maintain a high temperature. These temperatures can be as high as 104°! It is not a good idea to raise your body temperature that much. You could become so weak that you could drown, or the severe rise in body temperature could cause a pseudo-exacerbation. See the "Defining Multiple Sclerosis" section for more information.

If I have MS, can I get a flu shot?

Yes! Recent studies have shown no association between flu shots and MS relapses. According to the National MS Society's Medical Advisory Board, flu shots are safe for people with relapsing-remitting MS. But of course the decision is up to you and your physician. Ask your doctor for his or her opinion about your particular condition before getting a flu shot.

Should someone with MS rest?

Yes. Every person should find his or her comfort zone—the number and length of naps needed per week.

For the past few years after I was diagnosed, I was able to work full time as long as I took a nap on Saturday and Sunday. This year that changed for me. The two naps a week were not enough, so I cut my work hours to three days a week. Now, I work Monday, Wednesday, and Friday. I take a one- to two-hour nap on Tuesday, Thursday, Saturday, and Sunday.

During the summer, I nap almost every day. This can be a difficult undertaking if you have children. My children know that I need to rest, so we have quiet time at our house, during which they can play a computer game or read books in their room. I have found that if I don't take naps during the week or only have one nap, I can't function and end up missing a day of work. If you have young children who won't nap, you may need to ask a friend or hire a baby-sitter to watch them while you sleep.

Should someone with MS exercise? Will it help?

Absolutely! Exercise is good for everyone. It helps maintain a healthy heart, build strong bones and muscles, and increase strength and flexibility. It also lessens fatigue—all good reasons for someone with multiple sclerosis to exercise.

What exercises are recommended for people with MS?

Any that your doctor recommends and you enjoy doing! Here are a few suggestions:

- Pay attention to your body temperature during exercise. Don't get too overheated.
- Exercise in an air-conditioned room, if possible.
- Start out slowly and gradually work your way up to more intense exercises.
- Lifting weights, even in small amounts, is helpful for building strength.
- Stretching exercises such as yoga can help with stiffness and flexibility.
- Swimming or water aerobics is often recommended as a good choice for people with MS. You can regulate your own pace while building all-over body strength and toning, and stay cool!
- Walking is good for everyone. Just make sure that you walk during a cool part of the day, for example, early morning or evening. Don't get so far away from home that you are too fatigued to make it back! (Some people with MS carry a cell phone just in case!) Treadmills are not recommended for people who have balance and coordination problems.

- You might also want to consider a commercial cooling vest. A cooling vest is made with slots to hold long, thin ice or gel packs around your torso. Besides keeping you cool in the summer, these vests can also help keep your body temperature from rising during exercise.
- Finally, choose an activity in which you can set your own pace. There will be days when things go very well and you feel like Arnold Schwarzenegger (although not very many days). The majority of the time, you will probably feel like the eighty-year-old woman next to you on the weight machine is doing a better job than you! And she probably is. But, regardless, exercise is still good for you and it will help!

According to a study on MS by Dr. Jack Petajan, an MS specialist at the University of Utah, regular exercise improves strength, fitness, and bowel and bladder control, as well as reducing depression and fatigue. These are all good reasons to get started today!

Can I still drive?

Multiple sclerosis can cause numerous problems with driving and safety issues. These problems include: visual difficulties; fatigue; cognitive difficulties such as confusion, memory, and slower reaction times; and strength and stiffness issues.

Can you drive? If you physician says that you are able to drive and you pass the test from the Department of Motor Vehicles, then *legally* you are allowed to drive. Whether you feel comfortable driving is *another* issue. Night driving might be difficult or nearly impossible for you, and you might have trouble with glare or your peripheral vision.

But don't give up your keys yet. Many people with MS can continue to drive safely by making small adjustments in their routine and habits. Below are measures that you can take to ensure that you are driving safely:

- Don't drive when you are fatigued. Fatigue can cause your vision to blur.
- Stay cool. Use air-conditioning and bring a cold drink.
- Avoid high-speed roadways whenever possible.

- Some people can continue to drive by using vehicle modification devices.
- If you wear glasses, make sure your prescription is current and that it includes anti-glare provisions for night driving.
- Never drive when you are having an MS episode involving the eyes.
- Never drive when you are having an MS episode involving seizures—even short "absence" seizures.
- If the weather is bad, opt to stay home.
- Bring along a map, addresses, and phone numbers.
- Cell phones can be very useful if you are lost or if your car breaks down.
- When friends offer to drive, let them.
- Take other modes of transportation—buses, trains, and planes—for long journeys.
- To avoid muscular stiffness and pain, get out of the vehicle and stretch on a regular basis.
- Keep your car maintained.

Finally, keep in mind, if you feel that it is no longer safe for you to drive, you are probably right. Don't wait until an accident happens to quit driving. There are also numerous options for people who can't drive because of disability. These options include intercity bus lines, taxis, "Access Van" and "Dial-a-Ride," subways, carpooling, and sharing a ride with a good-hearted friend.

Can I drink alcoholic beverages if I have MS?

In my opinion, and from my conversations with others with MS, drinking alcoholic beverages is not a good idea for someone with multiple sclerosis. Alcohol can cause blurred or double vision, difficulty with walking and coordination, and dizziness and fatigue (among other symptoms). Since many of us with MS *already* have these symptoms, drinking alcoholic beverages can make them much worse than they already are. In addition, alcohol can interact negatively with some medications that are used to treat MS symptoms (such as drugs used to treat depression or fatigue).

Who should I tell that I have MS?

Before I answer this, I'll tell you a little story. When I was a child, I had an elderly aunt who would call every day. For some reason, I would always answer the phone, and the conversation would go like this: "How are you, Auntie?" "Oh, not so good. My hemorrhoids are hurting me"—or some other embarrassing condition that I really didn't want to hear about.

The truth is, when people ask, "How are you?" most of them don't really want to know. It is a familiar greeting of sorts. So I generally don't talk about my MS with anyone other than family members or close friends. If I need to talk about it, I will ask someone if it is okay if I talk about it.

In the beginning phases of MS, you might feel like telling everyone, or you might want to keep it quiet. Here are a few guidelines to help you in your decision on who to tell:

- Inform close family members (spouse, parents, children) as soon as possible. Keep the conversation on a positive note. Giving family members the opportunity to read a good book on MS or a brochure from the National Multiple Sclerosis Society can be helpful. Often family members are as in the dark about MS as you are. Learning about the disease can be reassuring.
- Inform a few close friends who can serve as support for you, both emotionally and physically. My friends not only listen to me, but they sometimes help with housework, child care, and accompanying me to medical tests such as MRIs. I couldn't survive without them.
- If you are dating, it is often wise to discuss the disease only after the relationship becomes more serious. Talking about the disease with everyone can be boring. However, if the disease is obvious, you might want to briefly explain why you use a cane, etc. If the relationship becomes serious, you should discuss how the disease could affect your future together.

- Whether you inform your employer or not is up to you and depends on your work environment. Some employers are very supportive, while others could become concerned about your ability to perform your responsibilities. If your MS is not obvious and has not affected your performance on the job, you might choose to say nothing. If you have missed work because of an attack or need special accommodations because of MS (such as special doorknobs or a workspace near a bathroom), it would be better to inform your employer. When they know you are really sick, employers are often more understanding than when they think you are just taking lots of time off work for no reason. In addition, other symptoms of MS, such as shakiness or tremor, can be confused with alcohol or drug abuse, and you don't want to give anyone the wrong idea.

Should I work?

This is a difficult question to answer, because no one knows what course MS will take for you. For example, you might have a few episodes and then the disease could quiet down, or the disease might take a steadily progressive course. It is also possible that the fatigue associated with multiple sclerosis could become disabling for you. How you feel can change daily. There might be times when you can perform your job easily and times when it is a struggle or downright impossible. Decisions about whether or not to work should not be made quickly. A condition that is severe today might completely clear up by next month.

Often, friends will advise you to quit and go on Social Security and Medicare, but the fact is that work is often beneficial to people, financially, physically, and psychologically. In some cases, changing careers or working part time can be a better option.

I work as a teacher and this year found that I could no longer work full time. I wasn't able to make it through the week and ended up missing a day of work to rest. So my husband and I met with my benefits representatives and decided that I should cut my hours back to 60 percent. Now I work three days a week: Monday, Wednesday, and Friday. I only work one day at a stretch, which is manageable for me. I have also kept my benefits by picking up 40 percent of the cost. We've taken a loss financially, but the amount I have gained physically and psychologically is phenomenal. I hope I'll be able to continue like this for a long time.

Should I quit my job?

This is a difficult question to answer. There are numerous factors you should think about, including the following:

- Do you have health insurance through your job? What would you do for health insurance if you quit? Could you afford private health insurance?
- Do you have prescription coverage through your work? Do you currently use one of the disease-modifying medications? Could you afford to pay for the disease-modifying medications on your own?
- Do you have disability insurance? What are the rules and regulations concerning your disability insurance? Is there a waiting period? How much of your salary will it cover? Will it provide benefits until you are sixty-five?
- Do you like what you do? Does your work make you feel fulfilled?
- Are you helping others in your everyday work? Do you feel that what you are doing is worthwhile or helpful to society?
- If you weren't working, what would you do with your time?
- Does the stress of your job affect your MS?
- Do you consistently use more than your allotted amount of sick days for flare-ups?
- Are you so fatigued that you can't participate in other activities outside of work?
- Can you afford to quit?
- Would your spouse have to work an extra job or overtime hours to make up for the loss of income if you quit?
- Can you cut back the number of hours you work or work part time?
- What is your age? How long have you worked at your current job?
- If you quit your job, would you be able to return if you wanted to? Would it be at a lower salary?

- Would you be in the same position or a different one? If your company wouldn't hire you back, could you get a position with another company?
- What about retirement? Do you have a retirement fund? What will you use for your retirement if you quit? Can you take early retirement?
- Would special provisions at your place of employment help you maintain your employment status? If so, what are they? Would your employer be willing to provide them for you?

According to the National Multiple Sclerosis Society, only 30 percent of those with MS are still working full time after twenty years. With the advent of the new drugs, however, this number might be changing in the near future.

Whether you work or how many hours you work is really a decision between you, your spouse, your doctor, and sometimes your employer. Some employers are very flexible when they find out that an employee has MS. Accommodations can be incorporated, such as giving you an office near a bathroom or installing special doorknobs and handles. In my work situation in the school where I teach music, my principal is very supportive. When I began having fatigue problems, she found a room that I could use as a music classroom rather than having to go from class to class with my music supplies in a cart. Flextime, working part time, and working from home are other possible options for a valuable employee with MS. Every situation is different.

Before making a decision, you should discuss the situation fully. You might also want to discuss your options with a financial adviser. Your local chapter of the National Multiple Sclerosis Society can also be helpful in this area. Note: If you quit your job and take a position with another company, insurance will often not cover preexisting conditions for a certain period. Please keep this in mind if you need to switch insurance providers for any reason.

Q Can my employer discriminate against me because of my MS?

Discrimination shouldn't happen, but sometimes it does. The Americans with Disabilities Act (ADA) serves to protect people with disabilities. According to the ADA, an employee must be able to perform their essential job functions, but nonessential functions should be given to other employees. Also, reasonable accommodations must be made for that employee. "Reasonable accommodations" could include accessible office space, accessible parking spaces, special equipment (such as doorknobs or ramps), and flextime. For advice on reasonable accommodations, call JAN (Job Accommodation Network) at 1-800-ADA-WORK or visit their website, janweb.icdi.wvu.edu. (The Job Accommodation Network is a service of the Office of Disability Employment Policy of the U.S. Department of Labor.) JAN's mission is to "facilitate the employment and retention of workers with disabilities by providing employers, employment providers, people with disabilities, their family members, and other interested parties with information on job accommodations, self-employment and small business opportunities, and related subjects."

Other Relevant Questions About Multiple Sclerosis

· ·

What is NARCOMS? Is it legitimate? Should I register?

NARCOMS (the North American Research Committee on Multiple Sclerosis) is a patient registry that was developed by a team of respected neurologists in the field of multiple sclerosis. Anyone who has been diagnosed with MS is eligible to participate in the registry. Information about MS patients is collected through a questionnaire twice a year—either by mail or through their secure Internet server. In the questionnaire, patients are asked about their medical history, symptoms, therapies, and medications used, as well as to rate themselves on a disability performance scale. More than twenty thousand people with MS currently participate in the registry. Besides helping scientists by providing important information about the disease, participants receive a copy of the *Multiple Sclerosis Quarterly Report*.

So, is it legitimate? Yes. It is supported by grants and services from the National Multiple Sclerosis Society, the Eastern Paralyzed Veterans Association, the Paralyzed Veterans Association, and Berlex, Biogen, Amgen, Serono, and Teva Neuroscience (the manufacturers of the disease-modifying medications). Should you register? Yes. It's free, it's confidential, it benefits you, and it promotes MS research. To register, visit the NARCOMS website at www.narcoms.org or contact the registry office at 1-800-253-7884. You can also reach them by email at narcoms@mscare.org.

What about the National Multiple Sclerosis Society? What can it do for me?

What can the National Multiple Sclerosis Society do for you? So much, I can hardly begin listing everything here! According to the NMSS website, the organization "supports more MS research and serves more people with MS than any other MS organization in the world." Here are just a few of the ways they help those with MS and their families lead more fulfilling lives through research, service, education, fund-raising and advocacy programs.

Research. Since the society was founded in 1946, they have invested more than $350 million in MS research. In 2001 alone, they invested $29 million to support more than three hundred researchers. These investments help bring about advances in treatments, as well as moving us closer every day to a cure!

Service. With a fifty-state network of chapters and divisions, the society services more than a million people annually! A few of their service programs include:

- Helping people with MS find and keep their jobs
- Providing accurate and up-to-date information about MS
- Free counseling
- Self-help groups
- Assistance with medical equipment
- Referrals to qualified medical professionals (For a list of National Multiple Sclerosis Society–affiliated clinics, see the appendix.)

Education. The National Multiple Sclerosis Society has the largest library on MS in the world. Just a few of their educational programs include:

- Numerous brochures on a multitude of topics dealing with multiple sclerosis
- *InsideMS* magazine
- *Teen InsideMS* magazine
- *Keep S'myelin,* a fun newsletter for five- to twelve-year-olds
- The "Knowledge Is Power" program for the newly diagnosed
- A comprehensive website located at www.nationalmssociety.org
- Local programs and conferences about MS-related issues
- "MS Learn Online," live broadcasts about MS (See the society's website, www.nationalmssociety.org, for more information.)

Fund-raising. In 2001, the National Multiple Sclerosis Society received $156 million in support from individual gifts, membership dues, special events, and corporate contributions. Locally, society chapters organize many different special events and campaigns to help raise these funds. Nationally, the top two fund-raising events are the MS 150 Bike Tour and the MS Walk. More than 250,000 people participate in these two events each year.

Advocacy. The National MS Society advocates for those with MS at the federal, state, and local levels. These policy areas include federal funding for MS research; disability rights; access to quality health care; access to adequate, fairly priced health insurance; and access to quality, appropriate, long-term care options.

As you can see, I am clearly a National Multiple Sclerosis Society fan and member, and I strongly encourage you to join. The National MS Society has been an incredible help to me in so many ways.

You can also be part of the fight against MS; 70 percent of your donation goes to the programs listed above. The National Multiple Sclerosis Society is, without a doubt, our best advocate in the fight against multiple sclerosis. For questions about the National Multiple Sclerosis Society or to join, call 1-800-FIGHT MS.

PART III

. . . .

SUGGESTIONS

. . . .

WHAT TO DO
IF YOU THINK YOU
HAVE MS BUT HAVEN'T
YET BEEN DIAGNOSED

. . . .

Without a doubt, one of the most frustrating aspects of having multiple sclerosis is getting a diagnosis and figuring out what to do until that time comes. Below are some things that I wish someone had told me when I was first experiencing symptoms. I hope they are helpful for you!

1. *Find a good primary-care physician, neurologist, and ophthalmologist, and stick with them.* Switching from doctor to doctor can delay your diagnosis. Often, a physician will need to observe the symptoms over time. He can't easily do this if he just met you. Also, getting into a specialist for the first time can sometimes take three months or more. Don't wait until you are having an attack to try to see someone. Have a relationship already established.

2. *Keep a record of your symptoms.* Record the date and time the symptom started and ended. Explain the symptom and how severe it was. Record any significant events that were taking place during the time of symptom (for example, an illness, a stressful situation, or an injury). Record any visits to your doctor, what was discussed, and the doctor's suggestions for treatment.

3. *Get a good health insurance policy, if you don't already have one, and make sure that it includes prescriptions.* Call and see if the disease-modifying medications Avonex, Betaseron, Copaxone, and Rebif

are covered under your policy. (At the time of this publication, these medications cost $1,200 a month.) See what the deductible is for prescriptions. Note: It is nearly impossible to get private health insurance after you have been diagnosed! Get it now!

4. *Get a good life insurance policy and an excellent disability policy.* If you are working, make sure that the disability policy would completely replace your salary. Note: It is nearly impossible to get either of these things after you have been diagnosed! (For more information, read Laura D. Cooper's book *Insurance Solutions, Plan Well, Live Better: A Workbook for People with Chronic Illnesses or Disabilities.*)

5. *Contact the National Multiple Sclerosis Society and get a free packet of information, or visit their website.* Many people suffer from MS for years before receiving a diagnosis. People who work or volunteer for the MS Society are familiar with this and can lead you in the right direction. You might also want to consider talking to someone from the NMSS about your situation. Other helpful organizations include the MS Association of America, the MS Foundation, and the Montel Williams MS Foundation.

Twenty Things to Do
if You Have MS

. . . .

1. Find a good neurologist and stick with him or her.
2. Research and choose one of the disease-modifying drugs (Avonex, Betaseron, Copaxone, or Rebif) and start using it ASAP.
3. Become a member of the National Multiple Sclerosis Society and sign up for their quarterly newsletter. If you are newly diagnosed, you should also ask for their "Knowledge Is Power" series. Other helpful organizations include the MS Association of America, the MS Foundation, and the Montel Williams MS Foundation.
4. Participate in the MS Walk to help raise money for research.
5. Visit the National Multiple Sclerosis Society's website monthly for new and updated information.
6. Join a health spa or work with your doctor to develop a good exercise program.
7. Eat a well-balanced diet and drink plenty of water.
8. Maintain a healthy weight.
9. Try to keep your stress level low.
10. Avoid overextending yourself.
11. Learn to accept the help of friends and family.
12. Rest more often and take naps!
13. Watch your body temperature (stay cool in the summer and avoid getting sick).

14. Register with NARCOMS.
15. If you are religious, pray every day, in the car, in the shower, whenever you can.
16. Be grateful for what you have.
17. Laugh! A sense of humor will get you through anything.
18. Don't give up hope.
19. Remember that a cure is coming in our lifetime.
20. Remember that you are not alone.

SUGGESTIONS
FOR FRIENDS OF
MS PATIENTS

. . . .

If someone you know has multiple sclerosis, you can be of great help
to them. Use the following ideas to help guide you.

1. Be compassionate. Say, "I'm sorry" and "Is there anything I can
   do to help?"
2. Don't use platitudes like "God never gives you more than you can
   handle" or "God gave you this because you are a special person."
3. Offer to help with housework or take care of her children for
   a while. Don't expect her to reciprocate. Sometimes it is easier
   for her to hire a baby-sitter than be expected to baby-sit for someone else.
4. Don't always ask him, "How are you feeling?" Your friend is more
   than his MS. He is still the same person you know and love. His
   MS is only a small part of his identity.
5. A small token can be nice at times. A piece of pie or some freshly
   picked flowers can always brighten someone's day.
6. Use humor. Making light of things can sometimes help everyone
   through a difficult moment.
7. Help get her out of her environment. An afternoon at the park or
   evening at a karaoke bar may just do the trick.

8. If your friend likes to exercise, offer to go with him. Or perhaps an afternoon as a spectator at a football or soccer game would be a better choice.

9. Listen when she needs to talk. Offer a shoulder to cry on.

10. Tell her that you are there for her.

SUGGESTIONS FOR THE SPOUSE OR SIGNIFICANT OTHER OF AN MS PATIENT

. . . .

When one member of the family has multiple sclerosis, everyone in the family has to learn to cope with the disease. It can affect and change many things in your family environment. It can change your roles as husband and wife, as parent, as breadwinner, as housekeeper, or as child-care provider. Below are a few suggestions to help you with these changes:

1. Be flexible. Be willing to change your family roles as the disease progresses.
2. Be available and willing to listen. Fear, frustration, and anger are common emotions when dealing with MS.
3. Go to doctor appointments with your spouse or significant other.
4. Educate yourself on the disease.
5. Don't assume that because she looks okay, she feels okay. MS is often invisible to everyone except the sufferer.
6. Pray together.
7. MS can make the difficulties of marriage or relationships even harder. Don't be afraid to get counseling.

8. Give your spouse or significant other opportunities to rest.
9. Tell him often that you love him.
10. Encourage playfulness and fun in your relationship. A picnic under the stars or some other simple activity can help refresh and revitalize your relationship.

CONCLUSION

· ·

This is the end of *Multiple Sclerosis Q&A*. I hope that this book has been of some help to you. You will have good days and difficult days in your battle against multiple sclerosis. It is a terrible disease. But you are more than your disease. You are mother, father, friend, husband, wife, employee, boss, and teacher. You are so much more. Remember, the cure is nearly upon us. Surely in our lifetime we will see it happen. You won't have this illness forever. The goal is to hold on, to postpone the damage to your body as long as possible, and to live a full and happy life. You are important. You are special. You are not alone. And remember, there is hope!

When I was a child, my grandfather used to tell me, "There are only two things you have to do in life—die and pay taxes!" Well, he was wrong. There is one more thing: You have to change. Our lives are constantly changing, and I know mine certainly did in September 1995, when I developed multiple sclerosis. That major change in my life was unexpected and I was afraid. And the question that kept popping into my head was "Why me?"

In her book *The Winning Spirit*, Zoe Koplowitz talks about "Why me?" I love her answer. "As for the ponderous philosophical question 'Why me?,' perhaps the answer was far simpler than I had suspected. Maybe the answer could be summed up in six letters. Two very simple words: 'Why not?' "

Why not me? Why not you? It's happened—a change that we never expected or anticipated. It's nobody's fault. Being angry and bitter won't help us. Experts say that there are certain stages that we go through in the grieving process: denial, anger, sadness, and, finally, acceptance. I don't think that we ever get to the acceptance part with multiple sclerosis. We never do accept that we have this terrible disease. I believe that we instead graduate to a stage called the "alright then" stage. We don't like the disease. It's not okay for it to be here. We don't accept it. Instead, we look in the mirror and we say, "All right then! Where do we go from here?" Maybe this should really be the question you ask yourself: "Where do I go from here?" And "What can I do with my life that is special and beautiful?"

Multiple sclerosis will change your life in a big way. It could change your health, your occupation, your family role, your relationships, and your ability to do some of the things that you enjoy. But maybe this isn't the change with which we should be concerned. Maybe the real change will be inside of us, and this is something that we have a lot of control over.

I have a student named Stephen. Stephen is eight years old and disabled. He is in a special education class at the school where I teach music. Stephen's head is misshapen. He has a disease that is expanding his head from the inside out. Someday, it will kill him. But you wouldn't know it to be around Stephen. His brown eyes shine with a love for life. And he loves music. He adores it. Every day that I come in, he sings a new song for me.

One day in music class, Stephen announced that he wanted to be a rock star when he grew up. Immediately, an image of perfect bodies swaying before a crowd of cheering fans flashed before me. Stephen would never be a rock star. As I was driving home, I thought about Stephen's dream. I thought about how unfair life was and what a sweet boy he is. And then, it dawned on me that perhaps my idea of a rock star and Stephen's were not one and the same.

The next day, I went to a costume store and bought ten pretend, inflatable instruments. When I got to Stephen's class, I made an announcement, "Today, we are going to be rock stars!" I gave Stephen a microphone and gave the other instruments to his classmates. Then I turned on his favorite CD, and away we went. We were rock stars. We were jamming. You never heard such beautiful music or saw a more enthusiastic crowd. And Stephen reached his dream. He was a rock star.

This is what we need to do with our multiple sclerosis. We need to think outside the box and change what is in our minds. One of my dreams has always been to visit the Grand Canyon—to ride a mule and experience the beauty of the canyon firsthand. But now, I don't have the strength and stamina for that kind of journey. And the heat would very quickly do me in. Then, I was reading an article in the summer 2001 issue of *InsideMS*. It was about how you could travel and still enjoy yourself. In this article was an idea about seeing the Grand Canyon by helicopter. I don't know about you, but that sounds more exciting than sitting on a mule! Much nicer and without the saddle sores.

That's what Stephen taught me. To think outside of the box. To not just assume that I can't do something now because I am ill. I may have to change my idea of what a rock star is. But I can still have the experience. To live hopefully ever after with multiple sclerosis, we must never give in. We must fight the disease and never accept that it has a home within us. Someday, we will be rid of it. Someday soon. Until that time, let's think outside of the box. If you can't play sports anymore—coach. If you can't work anymore, volunteer at your children's school or at a soup kitchen. Learn to play the piano or paint. There is so much that we can do to make our lives a lovely, sweet song—despite having multiple sclerosis.

All right then!

Appendix:

List of MS Clinical Facilities Affiliated with the National Multiple Sclerosis Society

Contact the national chapter of the National Multiple Sclerosis Society to find information about local chapters, events, helpful information, and resources.

National MS Society
773 Third Ave.
New York, NY 10017
www.nationalmssociety.org
1-800-FIGHT MS (1-800-344-4867)

The following clinical facilities have a formal affiliation with the National Multiple Sclerosis Society. The appropriate chapter clinical advisory committee, composed of MS experts, has reviewed and approved the affiliation. The following clinical facilities are listed by state.

ALABAMA

Neurology Department, UAB
The School of Medicine
University of Alabama at Birmingham
University Station
Birmingham, AL 35294
(205) 934-2402

CALIFORNIA

Cedars Sinai Medical Center, MS Treatment Center
8631 W. Third St., 1001 E. Tower
Los Angeles, CA 90048
(310) 423-2474
(310) 423-0148 (FAX)

Department of Rehabilitation, MS Clinic
Santa Clara Valley Medical Center
751 South Bascom Ave.
San Jose, CA 95128
(408) 885-2000

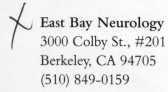

East Bay Neurology
3000 Colby St., #201
Berkeley, CA 94705
(510) 849-0159

Harbor–UCLA Medical Center, Multiple Sclerosis Clinic
1000 West Carson St.
Torrance, CA 90505
(310) 222-3897
(310) 533-8905 (FAX)

Kaiser-Permanente Medical Center
900 Kiely Blvd.
Santa Clara, CA 95051
(408) 236-4999

Loma Linda University Neurology Associates
Medical Group, Inc.
MS Clinic
11370 Anderson St., Suite 2400
Loma Linda, CA 92354
(909) 558-2120

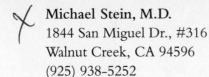

Michael Stein, M.D.
1844 San Miguel Dr., #316
Walnut Creek, CA 94596
(925) 938-5252

Mount Zion Multiple Sclerosis Center, UCSF
1600 Divisadero St.
San Francisco, CA 94115
(415) 885-7844

MS Comprehensive Care Center at USC University Hospital
1510 San Pablo St., Suite 268
Los Angeles, CA 90033-4606
(323) 442-6870
(323) 442-5773 (FAX)

Neurology Medical Group of Diablo Valley, Inc.
130 La Casa Via, #206
Walnut Creek, CA 94598
(510) 939-9400

The Northridge MS Center
18433 Roscoe Blvd., Suite 108
Northridge, CA 91326
(818) 349-2503

Parnassus MS Center
900 Parnassus Ave.
San Francisco, CA 94143
(415) 476-4173

Rancho Los Amigos Hospital
Division of Neurosciences
7601 East Imperial Way
Building 100, Clinic 1
Downey, CA 90242
(562) 401-7115 or (562) 401-7093
(562) 401-6247 (FAX)

Reed Neurological Research Center, UCLA
PO Box 951769
Los Angeles, CA 90095-1769
(310) 825-7313
(310) 206-9801 (FAX)

St. Mary's Hospital, MS Clinic
2200 Hayes St.
San Francisco, CA 94117
(415) 750-5762

Transitions Rehabilitation Multiple Sclerosis Clinic
7101 Monterey St., Suite A
Gilroy, CA 95020
(408) 842-6868

UCLA—Neurological Services
300 Medical Plaza, Suite B200
Los Angeles, CA 90024-6975
(310) 794-1195
(310) 794-7491 (FAX)

University of California
107 Irvine Hall
Irvine, CA 92717
(714) 824-5692

West LA VA Medical Center
11301 Wilshire Blvd.
Los Angeles, CA 90073
(310) 268-3891 or (310) 268-3013
(310) 268-4611 (FAX)

APPENDIX |

COLORADO

Denver Health Medical Center
Eighth and Bannock St.
Denver, CO

Saccomanno Education Center
St. Mary's Hospital
Grand Junction, CO

CONNECTICUT

Gaylord Hospital Multiple Sclerosis Clinic
PO Box 400
Wallingford, CT 06492
(203) 284-2845

West Haven–VAMC
Multiple Sclerosis Program
950 Campbell Ave.
West Haven, CT 06516
(203) 937-4735

Yale University School of Medicine MS Clinic
40 Temple St., Suite 7I
New Haven, CT 06510-8018
(203) 764-4280

FLORIDA

Baptist Medical Art Building—MS Clinic
8940 North Kendall Dr., Suite 802E
Miami, FL 33176
(303) 595-4041

Halifax Multiple Sclerosis Center
303 N. Clyde Morris Blvd. (201 Bldg.)
Daytona Beach, FL 32114
(904) 226-4506

Healthsouth Sea Pine Rehabilitation Hospital
101 East Florida Ave.
Melbourne, FL 32901
(407) 984-4600

MS Clinic
Healthsouth Rehabilitation
3251 Proctor Rd.
Sarasota, FL 34231
(941) 921-8600

Neurological Center
12901 Bruce B. Downs Ave.
Tampa, FL 33612
(813) 974-2722

North Florida Multiple Sclerosis Comprehensive Care Center
at St. Luke's Hospital
4203 Belfort Rd.
Rodget Main Building, Suite 115
Jacksonville, FL 32216
(904) 296-5731
(904) 296-4088 (FAX)

North Ridge Neuroscience Center
5757 North Dixie Highway
Ft. Lauderdale, FL 33334
(954) 928-0611

Orlando Regional MS Center
9430 Turkey Lake Rd., Suite 200
Orlando, FL 32819
(407) 351-8585

GEORGIA

Shepherd Center, Inc.
2020 Peachtree Rd., NW
Atlanta, GA 30309
(404) 350-7392

ILLINOIS

Central Illinois MS Center
Koke Mill Medical Center
3132 Old Jacksonville Rd.
Springfield, IL 62794
(217) 862-0422

Loyola University Medical Center MS Clinic
2160 South First Ave.
Maywood, IL 60153
(708) 216-6001

Northwestern Medical Faculty Foundation, Inc.
Department of Neurology
675 N. St. Clair St., Suite 20-100
Chicago, IL 60611
(312) 695-7950

Rush Presbyterian
St. Luke's MS Center
1725 West Harrison St., Suite 309
Chicago, IL 60612
(312) 942-8011

University of Chicago
The Duchossois Center for Advance Medicine
Room 4D
5758 Maryland Ave.
Chicago, IL 60637
(773) 702-6222

INDIANA

Caylor-Nickel Comprehensive MS Clinic
One Caylor-Nickel Square
Bluffton, IN 46714
(219) 824-3500 or (800) 756-2663

Indiana Center for MS
and Neuroimmunopathologic Disorders
8424 Naab Rd., #1A
Indianapolis, IN 46260
(317) 614-3100

Indiana University Multiple Sclerosis Center
541 Clinical Dr., Room 365
Indianapolis, IN 46202-5111
(317) 274-4030

Innovative Therapy Services
10601 N. Meridian St., Suite 110
Indianapolis, IN 46278
(317) 575-2100 (rehabilitative service)

IOWA

MS Center at Iowa Lutheran Hospital
700 E. University
Des Moines, IA 50316
(515) 263-5666

Physicians Clinic of Iowa, Neurology Department
600 Seventh St., SE
Des Moines, IA 52401
(319) 398-1721

Ruan Neurological Center
400 University Ave., West 5
Des Moines, IA 50314
(515) 643-4500

KENTUCKY

Baptist Hospital East
Neuroscience Associates
6400 Dutchmans Parkway, Suite 140
Louisville, KY 40205
(502) 895-7265

Frazier Rehabilitation Center
220 Abraham Flexner Way
Louisville, KY 40202-1887
(502) 582-7400

Purchase Area MS Clinic
225 Medical Center Dr., Suite 402
Paducah, KY 42002-8129
(502) 441-4400

University of Kentucky
Chandler Medical Center
Department of Neurology
Kentucky Clinic, L445
Lexington, KY 40536-0284
(606) 323-6702

University of Louisville
Department of Neurology
601 S. Floyd St., #503
Louisville, KY 40202
(606) 258-6830
(606) 258-6840 (FAX)

LOUISIANA

MS Clinic
Louisiana State University
2020 Gravier St., 7th Floor
New Orleans, LA 70112
(504) 568-4082

MS Clinic, Neurology Clinic
Tulane Medical Center
1415 Tulane Ave.
New Orleans, LA 70112
(504) 588-5231

MAINE

Maine Neurology, P.A.
49 Spring St.
Scarborough, ME 04074
(207) 883-1414

MARYLAND

Johns Hopkins Hospital
Department of Neurology
600 N. Wolfe St., Meyer 6-113
Baltimore, MD 21287-7613
(410) 955-5103

Maryland Center for MS Ambulatory
16 S. Eutaw St., Third Floor
Baltimore, MD 21201
(410) 328-5858

Total Rehab Care at Robinwood
1111 Medical Campus Dr., Suite 201
Hagerstown, MD 21740

University of Maryland
The School of Medicine
Department of Neurology
22 S. Greene St.
Baltimore, MD 21201
(410) 328-5605

MASSACHUSETTS

Metro West Medical Center
115 Lincoln St.
Framingham, MA 07101
(508) 879-1911

Mount Auburn Hospital
300 Mt. Auburn St., Suite 316
Cambridge, MA 02138
(617) 868-5014

Multiple Sclerosis Center
Brigham and Women's Hospital
Massachusetts General Hospital
333 Longwood Ave.
Boston, MA 02115
(617) 713-2030

MICHIGAN

Michigan State University
138 Service Rd.
A-217 Clinical Center
East Lansing, MI 48824
(517) 353-8122
(517) 432-3713 (FAX)

Mid-Michigan Regional Medical Center
4011 Orchard Dr., Suite 4010
Midland, MI 48640
(517) 835-8744
(517) 839-3369 (FAX)

Wayne State University
The School of Medicine
Department of Neurology
University Health Center, 6E
4201 St. Antoine
Detroit, MI 48201
(313) 745-4275
(313) 745-4468 (FAX)

West Michigan MS Clinic at Michigan Medical PC
3322 Beltline Ct., NE
Grand Rapids, MI 49525
(616) 456-9104

MINNESOTA

Fairview MS Center
Riverside Park Plaza
701 25th Ave. South, #200
Minneapolis, MN 55454
(612) 672-6100

The Minneapolis Clinic of Neurology, Ltd.
Golden Valley Office
4225 Golden Valley Rd.
Golden Valley, MN 55422
(612) 588-0661

Noran Neurological Clinic
910 E. 26th St., Suite 210
Minneapolis, MN 55404
(612) 879-1000

St. Luke's Hospital Trauma Center
915 E. First St.
Duluth, MN 55805
(218) 726-5555

SMDC—Comprehensive MS Program
400 E. Third St.
Duluth, MN 55805
(218) 725-3925

MISSOURI

Washington University MS Clinic
School of Medicine
Department of Neurology
Box 8111
660 South Euclid
St. Louis, MO 63110
(314) 362-3293

West County MS Center
St. John's Mercy Medical Center
621 S. New Ballas Rd.
Tower B, Suite 5003
St. Louis, MO
(314) 569-6933

NEBRASKA

University of Medical Associates
at the University of Nebraska Medical Clinic
600 S. 42nd St.
Omaha, NE 68198
(402) 559-7859

NEVADA

MS Service
50 Kirman Ave., #201
Reno, NV 89502
(775) 324-2234
(775) 324-6015 (FAX)

NEW JERSEY

Gimbel MS Center
718 Teaneck Rd.
Teaneck, NJ 07666
(201) 837-0727
(201) 837-8503 (FAX)

Kennedy Hospital at Statford
Voorhees Professional Building
102 White Horse Pike, Suite 101
Voorhees, NJ 08043
(856) 784-6800

RM Research and Treatment Center of UMDNY
185 South Orange Ave., H506
Newark, NJ 07103
(201) 982-2550

NEW MEXICO

University of Mexico
Department of Neurology
1201 Yale Blvd. NE
Albuquerque, NM 87131
(505) 272-3342
(505) 272-4056 (FAX)

NEW YORK

Bronx-Lebanon Hospital
1770 Grand Concourse
Bronx, NY 10457
(718) 960-1335

Buffalo General Hospital
100 High St.
Buffalo, NY 14203
(716) 859-7592
(716) 859-2430 (FAX)

Care Center at North Shore University
Hospital at Syosset
221 Jericho Turnpike
Syosset, NY 11791
(516) 727-0660

Columbia-Presbyterian Medical Center
MS Care Center
16 E. 60th St.
New York, NY 10022
(212) 326-8455

Columbia-Presbyterian Medical Center
MS Care Center, Vanderbilt Clinic
710 W. 168th St.
New York, NY 10032
(212) 305-5508

Department of Neurology
MS Clinic at SUNY Upstate Medical University
University Health Care Center
90 Presidential Plaza
Syracuse, NY 13210

Helen Hayes Hospital MS Clinic
Route 9W
West Haverstraw, NY 10993
(914) 947-3000

Hospital for Joint Diseases
301 E. 17th St.
New York, NY 10003
(212) 598-6305

Maimonides Medical Center
4802 10th Ave.
Brooklyn, NY 11219
(718) 283-7470

The New York Hospital–Cornell Medical Center
525 E. 68th St.
New York, NY 10021
(212) 746-4504

NY Hospital Medical Center, Queens MS Care Center
Department of Neurology
56-45 Main St.
Flushing, NY 11355
(718) 460-6765 or (718) 460-2903

St. Agnes MS Center
303 North St., Suite 203
White Plains, NY 10605
(914) 328-6410

St. Luke's–Roosevelt Medical Center
MS Treatment & Research Center
425 W. 59th St., Suite 7C
New York, NY 10019
(212) 523-8070

South Shore Neurologic Associates, PC
877 E. Main St.
Riverhead, NY 11901
(516) 727-0660

Staten Island University Hospital
Irving R. Boody Jr. Medical Arts Pavilion
475 Seaview Ave.
Staten Island, NY 10305
(718) 667-3800

Strong Memorial Hospital
University of Rochester
601 Elmwood Ave.
Rochester, NY 14642-8873
(716) 275-7854
(716) 442-9480 (FAX)

SUNY at Stony Brook
Department of Neurology
Health Science Center, T-12, Room 020
Stony Brook, NY 11790
(516) 444-1450

William C. Baird MS Research Center
Millard Fillmore Hospital
3 Gates Circle
Buffalo, NY 14209
(716) 887-5230
(716) 887-4285 (FAX)

NORTH CAROLINA

MS Center at Carolinas Medical Center
PO Box 32861
Charlotte, NC 28232-2861
(704) 446-1900

Triangle MS Center
Durham Clinic
3901 N. Roxboro Rd.
Durham, NC 27704
(919) 479-4140 x114

Triangle MS Center
Raleigh Neurology Associates
4207 Lake Boone Trail, Suite 200
Raleigh, NC 27607
(919) 782-3456

OHIO

Mellen Center U-10
Cleveland Clinic Foundation
9500 Euclid Ave.
Cleveland, OH 44195
(216) 445-6800

Ohio State University Medical Center
Department of Neurology
466 W. 10th Ave.
Columbus, OH 43210-1228
(614) 293-4964
(614) 293-6111 (FAX)

OREGON

OHSU MS Clinic
Department of Neurology, L226
Oregon Health Science University
3181 South West Sam Jackson Park Rd.
Portland, OR 97201
(503) 494-5759
(503) 494-7242 (FAX)

PENNSYLVANIA

Allegheny University MS Treatment Center
420 E. North Ave., Suite 206
Pittsburgh, PA 15212
(412) 359-8850
(412) 359-8878 (FAX)

Geisinger Medical Center
100 N. Academy Ave.
Danville, PA 17822-1405
(570) 271-6590

Health South Rehab of Reading
1623 Morgantown Rd.
Reading, PA 19607-9455
(610) 796-6328

Hospital of the University of Pennsylvania
3 West Gates Building
3400 Spruce St.
Philadelphia, PA 19104-4283
(215) 662-6565

Knobler Institute of Neurologic Disease
467 Pennsylvania Ave., Suite 108
Fort Washington, PA 19034
(215) 643-9045

Lehigh Valley Hospital
Neuroscience Research
1210 S. Cedar Crest Blvd., Suite 1800
Allentown, PA 18103
(610) 402-8420

Penn State Hershey Medical Center
500 University Dr.
Hershey, PA 17033
(717) 531-8692
(717) 531-4694 (FAX)

Temple University
Department of Neurology
Broad and Ontario St.
Philadelphia PA 19140
(215) 707-7847

Thomas Jefferson University
Neurology Department
1025 Walnut St., Suite 310
Philadelphia PA 19107
(215) 955-2468

University of Pittsburgh
811 Lillian Kaufman Building
3471 Fifth Ave.
Pittsburgh, PA 15213
(412) 692-4920
(412) 692-4907 (FAX)

SOUTH CAROLINA

Medical University at SC
171 Ashley Ave.
Charleston, SC 29425
(843) 792-3223
(843) 792-8626 (FAX)

TEXAS

Baylor Methodist International MS Center
6560 Fannin, Suite 1224
Houston, TX 77030
(713) 798-7707

Ben Taub Hospital MS Clinic
1504 Taub Loop
Houston, TX 77030
(713) 793-3100

UTAH

The School of Medicine
University of Utah
50 North Medical Dr.
Salt Lake City, UT 84132
(801) 585-6032 or (801) 581-4283

VERMONT

Fletcher Allen Health Care
Multiple Sclerosis Clinic
FAHC–UHC Campus
1 S. Prospect St.
Burlington, VT 05401
(802) 847–4589

VIRGINIA

DePaul Medical Center
MS Clinic
6161 Kemsville Circle, #315
Norfolk, VA 23505
(757) 461–5400 or (757) 889–5201

WASHINGTON

Holy Family Hospital
MS Center
5901 N. Lidgerwood, Suite 25B
Spokane, WA 99207
(509) 489–5019

Multiple Sclerosis Clinic
Overlake Hospital
1035 116th Ave. NE
Bellevue, WA 98004
(425) 688–5900
(425) 688–5912 (FAX)

Multiple Sclerosis Clinic
The School of Medicine
University of Washington
BB933 Health Sciences Bldg. (Box 356490)
Seattle, WA 98195-6490
(206) 543-7272
(206) 685-3244 (FAX)

WEST VIRGINIA

Charleston Area Medical Center
501 Morris St.
Charleston, WV 25301
(304) 346-2272

WISCONSIN

Center for Neurological Disorders
St. Francis Hospital
3237 S. 16th St.
Milwaukee, WI 53215
(414) 647-5305

The Marshfield Clinic, MS Clinic
1000 N. Oak Ave.
Marshfield, WI 54449
(715) 387-9115

Medical College of Wisconsin
Department of Neurology
Clinic at Froedtert
9200 W. Wisconsin Ave.
Milwaukee, WI 53226
(414) 454-5200

University of Wisconsin
Department of Neurology
Medical School
600 Highland Ave.
Madison, WI 53792
(608) 263-5448

Glossary

acupuncture: An ancient Chinese method of treatment in which fine needles are inserted into various parts of the body.

alternative therapies: Therapies that are outside the traditional practice realm of physicians, including massage and acupuncture.

amalgam: A material used as dental filling material by dentists.

aromatherapy: The use of essential oils for therapeutic purposes.

attack: The appearance of new MS symptoms, lasting more than twenty-four hours.

autoimmune disease: A disease in which the body's immune system attacks its own tissues, causing illness. Multiple sclerosis is thought to be an autoimmune disease.

Babinski reflex: A neurological indication of MS in which the big toe moves up rather than down when the side of the foot is stroked.

B-cell: A kind of white blood cell that makes antibodies.

central nervous system: Includes the brain, spinal cord, and optic nerves.

chelation therapy: A potentially dangerous or fatal therapy that uses intravenous injections of crystalline acid to remove heavy metals from the bloodstream.

chiropractic therapy: Physical manipulation of parts of the body.

corticosteroids: Medications, usually administered intravenously, to reduce inflammation during an MS episode.

demyelination: The destruction or loss of myelin in the brain, optic nerve, and spinal cord.

depression: Feelings of sadness and helplessness that don't go away.

diplopia: Double vision.

dysesthesias: Altered sensations, such as itching, burning, or a feeling of "pins and needles."

EEG (electroencephalograph): A machine that records a patient's brain waves.

erectile dysfunction: Difficulty achieving or maintaining an erection.

evoked potential test: Electrical studies designed to measure how quickly your brain picks up visual, auditory, and pain messages.

exacerbation: A worsening of current symptoms or disability.

fatigue: Severe tiredness.

flare-up: A worsening of current symptoms or disability.

frequency: The need to urinate, despite having voided recently.

girdle sensation: Tight, constricting feeling around the chest.

hesitancy: Delay in ability to urinate.

hyperbaric oxygen: Chamber used to deliver high concentrations of oxygen to a patient.

incontinence: The inability to control the time and place of urination.

intramuscular: Into the muscle, as in intramuscular injection involving a 1¼-inch needle.

intravenous (IV): Delivered by injection directly into the patient's vein.

lesions (or plaque): A spot or location in the brain, optic nerve, or spinal cord that indicates demyelination.

Lhermitte's sign: An electric-shock sensation brought on by flexing the chin toward the chest.

lymphocytes: A type of white blood cell. There are two types of lymphocytes: B-lymphocytes, or B-cells, produce antibodies and are manufactured in the bone marrow; and T-lymphocytes, or T-cells, are manufactured in the bone marrow, but mature in the thymus. Helper T-cells help B-cells produce antibodies. Suppressor, or killer, T-cells suppress the production of antibodies by B-cells.

massage therapy: Rubbing or kneading of parts of the body to aid circulation and relax the muscles.

megavitamin: A larger than normal dose of vitamins.

MRI (magnetic resonance imaging): A test that uses magnetic fields and radio waves to produce images of various areas in the body.

myelin: A soft, waxy coating, made up of fats and proteins, that surrounds and protects nerve fibers.

neurologist: A physician who specializes in disorders and diseases of the central nervous system.

nocturia: The need to urinate frequently during the night.

nystagmus: Jerky eye movements.

oligoclonal bands: An indicator of chronic inflammation found in cerebrospinal fluid. Approximately 90 percent of people with MS have an abnormal level of antibodies as indicated in a spinal tap.

oligodendrocytes: A type of cell that produces myelin.

optic neuritis: Damage to the optic nerve causing blurred vision, color blindness, blind spots, and pain. Can be caused by demyelination.

paralysis: Inability to move various parts of the body.

paresthesias: Pain.

paroxsymal itching: Unexplained intense itching.

paroxsymal symptoms: Brief MS episodes, lasting from a few seconds to less than twenty-four hours.

plaque (or lesions): A spot or location in the brain, optic nerve, or spinal cord that indicates demyelination.

pseudo-exacerbation: A worsening of symptoms caused by a high fever due to an infection.

reflexology: Therapy using massage and pressure to various parts of the foot.

relapse: The appearance of new MS symptoms, lasting more than twenty-four hours.

remission: A disappearance of disease symptoms.

sclerosis: From the word "sclerotic," sclerosis means scarring. Multiple sclerosis means "many scars" along the central nervous system.

spasticity: Involuntary stiffness and sudden movements or spasms.

spinal tap (or lumbar puncture): A procedure in which a small amount of spinal fluid is removed through a needle inserted into the lower back.

subcutaneous: Just under the skin, as in subcutaneous injection involving a ½-inch needle.

susceptibility: The odds or chance of getting multiple sclerosis. (For example, MS susceptibility is greater for women, Caucasians, and those raised in colder parts of the world.)

tai chi: Ancient Chinese system of meditative exercise.

T-cells: T-lymphocytes, or T-cells, are manufactured in the bone marrow, but mature in the thymus. Helper T-cells help B-cells produce antibodies. Suppressor, or killer T-cells, suppress the production of antibodies by B-cells.

tremor: Involuntary, rhythmic shaking of the muscles.

trigeminal neuralgia: Facial pain.

urgency: The inability to delay urination.

vertigo: A spinning sensation.

yoga: A meditation and exercise technique that promotes relaxation, flexibility, and strength.

References

PERIODICALS

"Autoimmunity May Play Role in Disease." *USA Today* 128 no. 2653 (October 1999): 15–16.

"Brain Imaging System." *Electronics Now* 69 no. 10 (October 1998): 23–24.

Quinn, Thomas C. "Editorials, Chlamydia Pneumoniae and Multiple Sclerosis: Innocent Bystander or Culprit?" *Annals of Neurology* 49 no. 5 (2001): 556.

Seppa, Nathan. "Herpesvirus Linked to Multiple Sclerosis." *Science News* (December 6, 1997): 356.

Siblerud, R. L., and E. Kienholz. "A Comparison of Oral Health Between Multiple Sclerosis Subjects with Dental Amalgams and Those with Amalgams Removed." *Journal of Orthomolecular Psychiatry* 14 no. 2 (1999): 93.

Stolberg, Sheryl Gay. "Trade Agency Finds Web Slippery with Snake Oil." *New York Times* (June 25, 1999): A16.

Travis, John. "MS Families: It's Genes, Not a Virus." *Science News* (September 16, 1995): 180.

BOOKS

Gold, Susan Dudley. *Multiple Sclerosis.* Berkeley Heights, N.J.: Enslow Publishers, 2001.

Koplowitz Zoe, with Mike Celizic. *The Winning Spirit: Life Lessons Learned in Last Place.* New York: Doubleday, 1997.

Kraft, George H., and Marci Catanzaro. *Living with Multiple Sclerosis.* 2nd edition. New York: Demos Medical Publishing, 2000.

Swiderski, Richard M. *Multiple Sclerosis through History and Human Life.* Jefferson, N.C., and London: MacFarland & Company, Inc., 1998.

BROCHURES

"Clear Thinking about Alternative Therapies," National Multiple Sclerosis Society brochure.

"Controlling Relapses," National Multiple Sclerosis Society brochure.

"Exercise as Part of Everyday Life," National Multiple Sclerosis brochure.

"Genes and MS Susceptibility," National Multiple Sclerosis Society brochure.

"The History of Multiple Sclerosis," National Multiple Sclerosis Society brochure.

"Hormones in Multiple Sclerosis," National Multiple Sclerosis Society brochure.

"Just the Facts," National Multiple Sclerosis Society brochure.

"Living with Multiple Sclerosis," National Multiple Sclerosis Society brochure.

"The Multiple Sclerosis Therapy Guide: A Patient's Resource," Copaxone brochure.

"Pregnancy," National Multiple Sclerosis Society brochure.

NEWS RELEASES

"Preliminary Study Results Suggest Benefit of the Monoclonal Antibody Antegren to Treat MS," news release, National Multiple Sclerosis Society website.

"Reports Indicate No Association Between Vaccinations and MS," news release, National Multiple Sclerosis Society website.

"Room-temperature Betaseron Available Nationwide," May 15, 2002, news release, Berlex Laboratories, Inc. website.

Resources

BOOKS

All of a Piece. Webster, Barbara D. Baltimore: Johns Hopkins University Press, 1989.

Alternative Medicine and Multiple Sclerosis. Bowling, Allen C. New York: Demos Medical Publishing, Inc., 2000.

Coping When a Parent Has Multiple Sclerosis. Cristall, Barbara. New York: Rosen Publishing Group, Inc., 1992.

Coping with Multiple Sclerosis. Burnette, Betty, and Rob Getvertz. New York: Rosen Publishing Group, 2001.

Employment Issues and Multiple Sclerosis. Rumrill, Phillip D., Jr. New York: Demos Medical Publishing, Inc., 1997.

Fall Down, Laughing. Lander, David L. New York: Tarcher/Putnam, 2000.

Insurance Solutions, Plan Well, Live Better: A Workbook for People with Chronic Illnesses or Disabilities. Cooper, Laura D., Esq. New York: Demos Medical Publishing, Inc., 2002.

Life Lessons and Reflections. Williams, Montel. Mountain Movers Press, 2000.

Living Beyond Multiple Sclerosis. Nichols, Judith Lynn. Alameda, Calif.: Hunter House, Inc., 2000.

Living with Multiple Sclerosis, 2nd edition. Kraft, George H., and Marci Catanzaro. New York: Demos Medical Publishing, 2000.

Me and My Shadow. Mackie, Carole. London: Aurum Press, 1999.

Meeting the Challenge of Progressive MS. Halper, June. New York: Demos Medical Publishing, Inc., 2001.

Multiple Sclerosis. Gold, Susan Dudley. Berkeley Heights, N.J.: Enslow Publishers, 2001.

Multiple Sclerosis Fact Book. Lechtenberg, Richard, M.D. Philadelphia: F. A. Davis Company, 1995.

Multiple Sclerosis: The Facts You Need. O'Conner, Paul, M.D. Willowdale, Canada: Firefly Books, 1999.

Multiple Sclerosis: A Guide for the Newly Diagnosed, 2nd edition. Holland, Nancy, T. Jock Murray, and Stephen C. Reingold. New York: Demos Medical Publishing, 2002.

Multiple Sclerosis: The Guide to Treatment and Management. Polman, Chris H., and W. Ian McDonald. New York: Demos Medical Publishing, Inc., 2001.

Multiple Sclerosis and Having a Baby. Graham, Judy. Rochester, Vt.: Inner Traditions International, Limited, 1999.

Multiple Sclerosis: New Hope and Practical Advice for People with MS and Their Families. Rosner, Louis J., M.D., and Shelley Ross. New York: Simon & Schuster, 1992.

Multiple Sclerosis: Questions and Answers. Barnes, David. West Palm Beach, Fla.: Merit Publishing International, 2000.

Multiple Sclerosis: The Questions You Have—The Answers You Need, 2nd edition. Kalb, Rosalind C., Ph.D. New York: Demos Medical Publishing, 2000.

Multiple Sclerosis through History and Human Life. Swiderski, Richard M. Jefferson, N.C., and London: MacFarland & Company, Inc., 1998.

Multiple Sclerosis: Your Legal Rights, 2nd edition. Perkins, Lanny, and Sara Perkins. New York: Demos Medical Publishing, Inc., 1999.

Mysterious Stranger Aboard: A Couple's Courageous 40-Year Battle with Multiple Sclerosis. Johnson, Alice. Miami: Mal-Jonal Productions, 1995.

Reversing Multiple Sclerosis: 9 Effective Steps to Recover Your Health. Pepe, Celeste, and Lisa Hammond. Charlottesville, Va.: Hampton Roads Publishing Company, Inc., 2001.

Symptom Management in Multiple Sclerosis. Schapiro, Randall T., M.D. New York: Demos Medical Publishing, Inc., 1998.

300 Tips for Making Life with Multiple Sclerosis Easier. Schwarz, Shelley Peterman. New York: Demos Medical Publishing, Inc., 1999.

When the Road Turns: Inspirational Stories About People with MS. Russell, Margo. Deerfield Beach, Fla.: Health Communications, Inc., 2001.

The Winning Spirit: Life Lessons Learned in Last Place. Koplowitz Zoe, with Mike Celizic. New York: Doubleday, 1997.

You Are Not Your Illness: Seven Principles for Meeting the Challenge. Noble, Linda, Hal Topf, and Zina Bennett. New York: Simon & Schuster, 1995.

PERIODICALS, POPULAR MAGAZINES, AND NEWSPAPER ARTICLES

"Accessing the ABCs." King, Martha. *Inside MS* (Winter 2000): 50.

"Allied forces." Rudolph, Illeane. *TV Guide* (December 11–17, 1999): 42–43.

"The answer is in the bees." *Yankee* (August 1997): 48–51.

"Autoimmunity may play role in disease." *USA Today* (October 1999): 15–16.

"The billionaire and the orphan drug." Goldman, Lea. *Forbes* (October 2, 2000): 168–69.

"Brain-imaging system." *Electronics* (October 1998): 23–24.

"The challenge of his life." Sanz, Cynthia. *People* (October 16, 1995): 169–71.

"A comparison of oral health between multiple sclerosis subjects with dental amalgams and those with amalgams removed." Siblerud, R. L., and E. Kienholz. *Journal of Orthomolecular Psychiatry* 14 no. 2 (1999): 93.

"Conjugal multiple sclerosis: population-based prevalence and recurrence risks in offspring." Ebers, G. C., I.M.L. Yess, A. D. Sadovnick, and P. Duquette. *Annals of Neurology* 48 no. 6 (2000): 927–31.

"A cowboy's toughest ride." Day, Carol. *People* (September 29, 1997): 48.

"Developments to watch. How the brain spots faces, new hope for multiple sclerosis via cell grafts, love in the time of computer chips." *Business Week* (January 20, 1997): 91.

"A dream is a wish your heart makes." Cerio, Gregory. *People* (October 23, 1996): 111–12.

"Editorials, Chlamydia pneumoniae and multiple sclerosis: innocent bystander or culprit?" Quinn, Thomas C. *Annals of Neurology* 49, no. 5 (2001): 556–57.

"Feelings about assisted suicide." Cohen, Rose. *Inside MS* (Winter 2000): 47.

"A fighting chance." Schindehette, Susan. *People* (November 29, 1999): 150–54.

"Fighting multiple sclerosis. More young women than you think are battling this mysterious disease." *Cosmopolitan* (April 1, 1996): 162.

"A gender gap in autoimmunity." Whitacre, Caroline C., Stephen Charles Reingold, and Patricia A. O'Looney. *Science* (February 26, 1999): 1277–78.

"Glutamate glut linked to multiple sclerosis." Seppa, Nathan. *Science News* (January 8, 2000): 22.

"Herpesvirus linked to multiple sclerosis." Berardelli, Phil. *Science* (December 5, 1997): 1710.

"Herpesvirus linked to multiple sclerosis." Seppa, Nathan. *Science News* (December 6, 1997): 356.

"High flyer." Mackie, C. *We* (September/October 1999): 20.

"How I saved my own life." Kilcoyne, Colleen. *American Health* (March 1999): 104–5.

"I refuse to give in to a disabling disease." Hudepohl, Dana. *Glamour* (May 2000): 82–86.

"I will be there for you." Koplowitz, Zoe, and Mike Celizic. *Reader's Digest* (August 1998): 129–33.

"Incidental heroes." Gunkel, Gina Minielli, and Jackie Girsky Popper. *We* (March/April 2000): 64–69.

"The influence of cognitive impairment on driving performance in multiple sclerosis." Schultheis, M. T., E. Garay, and J. DeLuca. *Neurology* 56 no. 8 (2001): 1089–93.

"Learning from suffering." Mairs, Nancy. *The Christian Century* (May 6, 1998): 481.

"Let me tell you about picking up the pieces." Wright, Bret R. *Inside MS* (Winter 2000): 62.

"MS families: it's genes, not a virus." Travis, John. *Science News* (September 16, 1995): 180.

"MS sufferers seek out Md. woman for unorthodox bee-sting treatments." (August 19, 1993): Knight-Ridder/Tribune News Service.

"My doctor duped me." MacFarlane, Ellen. *Ladies' Home Journal* (January 1996): 36.

"A new look at MHC and autoimmune disease." Ridgway, William M., Marcella Fasso, and C. Garrison Fathman. *Science* (April 30, 1999): 749.

"On the job with MS." Huebner, Carol. *Inside MS* (Winter 2000): 12.

"One MS patient chose suicide; another chose to keep living." Garcia, Malcolm. (March 30, 1999): Knight-Ridder/Tribune News Service.

"Out of hiding." Lambert, Pam. *People* (June 14, 1999): 75–76.

"Planning for unplanned retirement." Perkins, Lanny, and Sara Perkins. *Inside MS* (Winter 2000): 19–22.

"Post mortem." *People* (September 16, 1996): 52–55.

"Pumping life into limbs." Winreb, Herman. *Prevention* (October 1996): 51–52.

"Researchers study Kevorkian deaths. Just 25 percent of those who sought Dr. Death were terminally ill." (December 7, 2000): Associated Press.

"Review—multiple sclerosis: the importance of early recognition and treatment." Fox, R. J., and J. A. Cohen. *Cleveland Clinic Journal of Medicine* 68 no. 2 (2001): 157–70.

"Rx for MS." Lindsey, J. William. *Prevention* (June 1997): 145.

"Singing praise." *People* (December 8, 1997): 115.

"Special article, clinical research, seizures in multiple sclerosis." *Epilepsia: The Journal of the International League Against Epilepsy* 42 no. 1 (2001): 72–79.

"Study of brains alters the view on path of MS." Kolata, Gina. *New York Times* (January 29, 1998): A1.

"A therapeutic bee sting?" Cerrato, Paul L. *RN* (August 1998): 57.

"Trade agency finds Web slippery with snake oil." Stolberg, Sheryl Gay. *New York Times* (June 25, 1999): A16.

"Transient symptoms in multiple sclerosis." Rae-Grant, Alexander D. *MSQR* Winter 2001: 10–12.

"When your nerves can't communicate." Rosenfeld, Isadore, M.D. *Parade Magazine* (May 20, 2001): 12.

"Who's calling?" Mairs, Nancy. *The Christian Century* (December 10, 1997): 1167.

"With faith to carry on." Osmond, Alan. *People* (June 19, 1995): 73–74.

"Wyrd made flesh." Mairs, Nancy. *The Christian Century* (January 21, 1998): 61.

NATIONAL MULTIPLE SCLEROSIS SOCIETY BROCHURES

Clear Thinking about Alternative Therapies: Facts and common misconceptions, comparison of alternative and complementary medicines, and suggestions on evaluating benefits and risks. By Virginia Foster.

Controlling Spasticity: Ways to control this common and sometimes disabling MS symptom. Includes roles of self-help, medications, physical therapists, nurses, and physicians. By Nancy Holland, R.N., Ed.D., with Serena Stockwell.

Hiring Help at Home?: Checklists and worksheets for people who need help at home, including forms for needs assessment, job description, and employment contract.

Keep S'myelin: A full-color newsletter for children ages five to twelve. Contains articles, interviews, games, and activities, and a special pull-out section for parents. Published four times a year. Request subscription from local chapter.

MS and the Mind: A colorful reprint from *InsideMS* on depression, cognitive functions, emotions, coping tips, and medications.

Overcoming Speech Problems: How speech problems can be helped with exercise, medications, or technological aids.

Stretching for People with MS: Illustrated manual provides basic range-of-motion, stretching, and balance exercises for at-home program. By Beth E. Gibson, P.T.

Vision Problems: Current therapy for MS-related eye disorders, plus discussion of low-vision aids.

The Win-Win Approach to Reasonable Accommodations: Enhancing Productivity on Your Job: A practical guide to obtaining workplace accommodations. By Richard T. Roessler, Ph.D., and Phillip Rumrill, Ph.D.

WEBSITES

American Chronic Pain Association: www.theacpa.org

Avonex: www.avonex.com

Betaseron: www.betaseron.com and www.mspathways.com

Copaxone: www.copaxone.com and www.mswatch.com

International Federation of Multiple Sclerosis Societies: www.msif.org

Job Accommodation Network (JAN): janweb.icdi.wvu.edu

The Mayo Clinic: www.mayoclinic.com

The Montel Williams MS Foundation: www.montelms.org

MS Awareness Foundation: www.msawareness.org

The MS Foundation: www.msfacts.org

Multiple Sclerosis Association of America: www.msaa.com

The Myelin Project: www.infosci.org/Myelin-Project

National Family Caregivers Association: www.nfcacares.org

National Multiple Sclerosis Society: www.nationalmssociety.org

North American Research Committee on Multiple Sclerosis (NARCOMS): www.narcoms.org

Novantrone: www.novantrone.com

Rebif: www.rebif.com

Trigeminal Neuralgia Association: www.tna-support.org

Index